ALPHA
BRAIN WAVES

ALPHA
BRAIN WAVES

David Boxerman and Aron Spilken

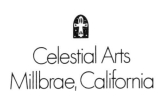

Celestial Arts
Millbrae, California

First Printing, May 1975
Made in the United States of America

Library of Congress Cataloging in Publication Data

Boxerman, David.
    Alpha brain waves.

    Bibliography: p.
    Includes index.
    1. Biofeedback training. 2. Alpha rhythms.
I. Spilken, Aron, 1939–   joint author. II. Title.
BF319.5.B5B69   152.1'88   74-25828
ISBN 0-89087-016-0

CONTENTS

   I. Alpha: The Wave of the Future   1

  II. What Is Alpha?: The Basic Facts   7

 III. The Coming of Alpha 27

 IV. A Matter of Life and Death 43

  V. Alphacare 57

 VI. The Followers of Alpha 63

VII. Building Your Own Biofeedback Machines 79

     Bibliography 103

     Index 109

ACKNOWLEDGMENTS

Grateful acknowledgment to Mitchell Waite for allowing us to use his excellent EEG biofeedback monitor circuits and for clarifying many technical details throughout; to Gary Mills, Ph.D., for technical assistance and most generous use of his time and energy; to Stanley Koehler for spiritual guidance at the inception of this project and thereafter; to Dennis Kaplan for his invaluable technical assistance and research.

DEDICATION

To Yvonne and Aaron

ALPHA
BRAIN WAVES

1

Alpha: The Wave of the Future

Introduction

The old man's pulse began to drop steadily. Alarmingly! The rate of his blood-flow diminished. His breathing became so shallow and slow that it would have been almost undetectable if it were not for the measuring instruments. All indicators pointed to impending death. No one lifted a finger to help.

Thousands in the audience watched the serene, aged face and wondered if he would die. Most of them must have also wondered if this were some kind of trick. Not only was this wrinkled Oriental operating at a physiological level which was believed unable to support life, but he was also locked in an airtight chamber holding barely enough oxygen for ten minutes. He had been in there for more than twenty minutes already. If he had been wired to measure the electrical activity of his brain, the machine would have shown a steady succession of smooth, slow, rhythmic waves: *Alpha.*

Suddenly he raised a finger as a signal that the trance was over. Physiological measures began to rapidly return to normal. Technicians raced frantically to undo the clamps securing the airtight box. With return to accelerated functioning in that stale, exhausted air he could not be expected to remain conscious for more than seconds. The alpha rhythms from his brain would be fading rapidly now, replaced by the more rapid, jagged and irregular patterns of normal alertness. Suddenly the door opened and the old man breathed deeply as the fresh air rushed in, still calm and apparently unconcerned about his voluntary brush with death. The doctors smiled with relief and congratulated each other on the successful experiment and the fascinating possibilities it suggested. At home, the thousands in front of their television sets wondered: What was this really all about? Was it just what it seemed? Did it have anything to do with me?

What they had seen was a Buddhist monk demonstrating that in a meditation-trance he was capable of controlling such mysterious bodily processes as heart rate, blood pressure, the entire speed of his metabolism. Because he was able to slow the rate at which his body used energy he was able to survive, conscious and with no ill effects, on less than half the normal amount of oxygen. This ability was not developed as a trick to inspire the unfaithful, but was a by-product of meditation skills which are claimed to grant those who master them enormous control over their minds as well as bodies, to refresh and give renewed spiritual vigor in meeting the difficulties of life, and to provide creative solutions to the most difficult problems.

One of the keys to this whole process may be the production of alpha waves in the brain. The recognition by Western scientists in the past few years that this mysterious and little understood knowledge was a fact and not a myth, and that it has been practiced in many parts of the world for thousands of years, has helped spark a whole new industry, radically changed traditional attitudes toward bodily functioning and the control of illness, suggested new approaches to learning, problem solving and creativity, and may permanently alter the philosophical base of our culture. And then again it may not. It will all depend on the outcome of experiments in process right now in hundreds of laboratories across the country.

Unlikely? Perhaps another scientific curiosity for researchers in university ivory towers to play with, but not something which will ever effect the average man-on-the-street? *Time* magazine noted in a recent article, "Defense Department researchers are said to be toying with the idea that captured U.S. intelligence agents trained to turn on alpha could foul up enemy lie dectors and keep military secrets. In industry, major companies are investigating biofeedback training to spur creative thinking and reduce executive tension." In typical American fashion every marketable or practical application of this new set of techniques will be explored and utilized, some very far indeed from the uses envisioned by the original Zen masters.

What are alpha waves? What are brain waves altogether, with their enigmatic Greek names? Where do they come from and what can they do? What about the new machines which claim to train one to control them, to "telescope up to 15 years of Zen meditation into a few easy hours"? What about the 150 people who paid $150 each (a total of $22,500 for four days of instruction in how to produce alpha without machines? They were hoping to learn how to use alpha to solve everyday problems, build confidence and develop healing Extra Sensory Perception—ESP. These courses are given regularly in many large cities and there is usually a waiting list of people who are fighting to get in.

What are the implications for big business in this new and mysterious area? Is there money to be made and if so how much and by whom? The *Wall Street Journal* reports that Xerox Corporation and Martin Marietta Corporation are already beginning to experiment on their own in order to get in on the ground floor. They are, however, mysteriously reluctant to discuss exactly what they are doing at this time. The same article mentions that the number of scientific researchers in the area has jumped from a small handful to more than 150 in the last three years and that there are already at least half a dozen private companies selling commercial machines to the general public now. "False hopes," they go on to warn, "seem to be one of the few risks of biofeedback training. 'Many people are buying machines—mostly the cheaper alpha trainers—in the belief that they are overnight-wonder-workers,' says one psychiatrist. 'But about the only real danger in that is that if it becomes a fad, a lot of gullible people will get fleeced.'" This concern is shared by a number of responsible workers in the field. "The propensity for exaggeration about progress in this area frightens prudent scientists. Already they are encountering the con-artists, the charlatans, and the quacks who are taking people's money by glibly mouthing the jargon associated with biofeedback research and similar studies of the mind's control over internal organs," as reported by *Saturday Review*.

But is "getting fleeced" to the tune of a few hundred dollars the only danger to the general public? At the Rockefeller University, rats which were used as subjects in biofeedback experiments to determine whether heart rate could be controlled (pioneer experiments which led the way to using human subjects with heart problems) learned to slow their heart rates so well they died! Are there dangerous consequences from tampering with the natural state of brain waves?

Descriptions of what the alpha state feels like have varied considerably and some reports have generated a great deal of enthusiasm or concern, depending on one's point of view. On the one hand there have been claims of individuals having a "dramatic reaction" when they first learn to control their brain waves. *Glamour* tells us, "They come out of the little room... looking positively radiant and report that they feel centered and open and free." Different people feel different things, reports another researcher. Some seem to feel high, like they have had a marijuana experience, while others just kind of slow down. On the other hand, Dr. Joseph Kamiya of Langley Porter Neuropsychiatric Institute in San Francisco claims that there aren't any psychedelic overtones to the alpha state. Why then has alpha training been mentioned as having a real potential in the treatment of drug addiction? Is there now a safe, legal and nonaddictive way to produce the euphoria and altered state of consciousness commonly called a high? Is there any possibility that the alpha party will replace the pot party?

The finding that certain types of individuals produce alpha more readily has led to some interesting speculation. Not only Zen masters, but also athletes, musicians and sensitive and introspective people tend to have greater access to alpha than the rest of the population. Is this somehow related to their exceptional abilities? Imagine what goes through the mind of a Gary Player just before sinking a putt which may be worth thousands of dollars. Is it alpha? The ability to invoke the relaxed awareness of the alpha state at critical moments, rather than choking up with tension, may be one of the talents which distinguishes the great man in any field.

Perhaps the greatest potential significance of current research into alpha (and the more generally encompassing area of biofeedback training) lies in its relationship to healing. It has been referred to as the most promising advance ever to occur in the field of psychology. Reliable researchers (although admittedly in their more effusive and speculative moments) consider it likely that current study in this area will lead to improved treatments for asthma, stroke, cancer, multiple sclerosis, cerebral palsy, migraine and muscle tension headaches, ulcers, warts, essential hypertension, numerous cardiac problems, stuttering and hyperactivity in children, obesity, alcoholism, drug addiction, insomnia, constipation, criminality and last, but not least, anxiety, depression and sexual problems. Unlikely? It's hard not to be skeptical of a list that sounds like an advertisement for snake oil. But many of the items mentioned above are currently being investigated by reputable scientists and many have already shown results which are encouraging and intriguing.

In addition to the hard facts about science and business there is another fascinating aspect of the alpha phenomenon which is part of a larger picture. When the chance to acquire new and special powers, the opportunity to become the leader in a new field, and the possibility of making a lot of money all meet at a single point, a varied and quite interesting group of people collect and try to speed or push their way to the center of power. Some may be altruistic, some egoistic, and some just seeking the promised relief from acute suffering. Together, however, they form a pattern also worth studying. The personalities of the individual scientists, salesmen, inventors, spiritualists, converts and skeptics all combine to produce a unique flavor, coloring and tone. The study of these people is satisfying just for what it tells us about human nature.

Let us look at the matter abstractly for a moment. A new possibility has occurred to the collective awareness of man: a promise that he can control inner forces in his nature as never before and unleash new potentials. Let us call it alpha. The vision is essentially messianic. It promises to provide guidance for one's life, to promote peace, love and wisdom. What is even better, it can be sold and promises to make the quick and the clever wealthy. It has all the aspects of that particularly American religion, a fad, and unlike traditional religions it has sprung up completely within our recent memory. Perhaps this time we can see it all happen.

We have seen the radiant faces of the new disciples, the unctuous paternalism of the pitchmen, and the fevered paranoia of the researcher rushing to publish before his colleagues. A mild-mannered scientist has been pushed into seclusion by unwanted notoriety. And another brushes off the alpha mania with good-natured humor. Companies file bitter suits against each other for the theft of ideas while selling peace and love to their customers. The prospect of greater wisdom for man prompts secret research in foreign countries and our own Defense Department. They all affect each other, and they may come to affect all of us.

2

What is Alpha?: The Basic Facts

Alpha waves are rhythms of electrical activity produced by the brain. In recent years scientists have been amazed to discover that under the proper conditions these natural processes and many others thought to be automatic and involuntary can actually be controlled by human and animal subjects. This has been occurring for thousands of years without anyone knowing about it, in those who became skilled in the practice of meditation. Many individuals who learn to produce large amounts of alpha waves report that they experience a pleasant euphoria or "high." Lately many claims about the effect of controlling brain waves have also been made. Interesting scientific findings have been accumulating rapidly. To understand and evaluate them reasonably you will have to know a bit about how the brain works and how scientists study it.

The brain is the hub of the nervous system, a communication network which functions much like a telephone company in a city. Messages are sent from one part of the body to another enabling it to carry out its work. While the analogy is quite simple the reality is awesomely complex. There are between 10 and 12 billion nerve cells in your body. They are carrying thousands upon thousands of messages to your brain simultaneously, at this very moment. Your attention can be focused on only a few of them at one time: the feel of this book in your hands; the patterns of the letters on the pages. But much, much more is going on, automatically, without conscious effort on your part, and with a degree of accuracy which is amazing. If your nervous system functioned no more efficiently than the telephone company you would be very sick indeed.

Take the page in front of you. Patterns of light and dark on a piece of paper are being analyzed by your brain into letters, words and finally meanings. Related meanings are also being pulled from your memory banks as needed to help you decide what you think about what you are reading. And all this is just a small part of what is happening now. The outer fringes of your awareness are constantly scanning your environment for other events of importance which might interrupt your reading: Is it safe where you are? Is it comfortable?

And still your brain is not nearly done because if you were able to read this far then your whole body with its trillions of cells and many organ systems is running smoothly enough to allow you to do something so unimportant (from the point of view of biological survival) as read about your brain. For no matter how much you read about your brain you are never likely to touch it, will not be able to fix it if it breaks, and neither you nor anyone else is likely to understand it well within your lifetime. The first lesson about the brain is ignorance. It knows what it is doing quite well. We don't.

We do know some things, however. We know that the nervous system produces its own faint electrical current like a battery does. The nerve cells, like telephone lines, transmit electric impulses which somehow allow the messages to be delivered. As early as 1791 Galvani found he could make the muscles in a frog's leg contract by applying a simple electrical current. Yet it was not until a hundred years later that electrical potentials in the brain were measured. One of the main reasons for this lag in progress was technological. For years there were no instruments to accurately measure the subtle electrical changes that took place within our bodies. Research on other organs with mechanical functions, such as the heart and lungs, proceeded steadily while our "electrical system" remained a mystery.

The Electroencephalograph

In the twentieth century the study of nerve function began to accelerate, as did most branches of science, with a tremendous boost from the technological explosion. One of the advances which contributed to this progress was the electroencephalograph. The large and cumbersome name fits a complex and expensive machine, but it only means that it supplies a written record (graph) of the electrical activity of the brain. It is usually abbreviated EEG. The EEG is important here because it is the primary method for studying brain waves.

In 1924, Neminski had shown that when he placed electrodes directly on the surface of the brain he recorded electrical waves of 10 to 15 cycles per second. Neminski's technique was obviously not suited for home use or repeated sessions of alpha wave training, however. It was not long after that Hans Berger, a German scientist considered to be the father of EEG science, found that electrical waves from the brain could be picked up from the scalp without having to open the skull. This was more practical, but not much. The basic clinical EEG machine still costs around $6500. The cost is prohibitive and it requires the services of a highly skilled technician, both to run and to interpret. It was not until the development of the alpha training machine in the last few years that exploration of brain potentials became practical for the average person.

The alpha machines on the market today cost in the neighborhood of $200 and are designed for use by the non-expert. They are simplified and specialized versions of the

EEG. A further understanding of that instrument will give greater skill in understanding the problems of home alpha recording.

The EEG is most commonly used to investigate brain functioning (research) and to measure abnormalities in the brain's behavior which might show the extent of an injury or the presence of a disease (diagnosis). If an abnormality is present the EEG sometimes helps "localize" it, or point out the exact location without the need for exploratory surgery, saving the patient from much additional danger. Its advantages and disadvantages stem from the same basic fact: It operates from outside the skull. Because it works through layers of blood vessels, fluids, skin and bone, it obtains its basic information without exposing the brain but it also sacrifices a certain amount of power and accuracy. About two-thirds of the voltage is lost because of this. The alpha machine has the same advantages and suffers from the same problems.

The currents which come from the brain are exceedingly weak. They are measured in millionths of a volt. Only those which come from the surface of the brain, or cortex, can be picked up. Diseases of the underlying brain tissue often remain hidden from the EEG. The same holds for healthy processes which may be of interest. Your alpha machine will tend to read off the top. The major portion of activity deep within your brain will not be detected. To obtain an EEG reading the technician will attach sensitive electrodes (wires) to the scalp. To increase their sensitivity small gold or silver plates are commonly attached to the ends which are glued down with electrode paste, or alternatively, the electrodes end in tiny needles which are inserted into the scalp. The procedure is not as painful as it sounds but may produce mild discomfort. Electrode paste is a glue which is also a good conductor of electricity. It helps hold the electrodes in place and insure good contact with the scalp. The subject is either lying down or leaning back in a comfortable chair and tries to remain as motionless as possible. This is extremely important since muscle movements also give off electrical potentials and the muscle signals, coming from just beneath the skin and not having to penetrate a layer of bone, are much stronger than the brain waves. They can override and mask the brain potentials in the EEG recording so attempts are made to filter them out.

With an EEG a permanent record is needed for detailed study. To provide this a paper tape is run through the machine and as many as 12 pens record the electrical signals from pairs of electrodes placed around the skull. The pens wave back and forth as the paper moves. Each rise and fall of the pen is one cycle. The paper moves at a constant rate of speed and is marked off in time units such as seconds. The electroencephalographer studies such characteristics of the waves as cycles per second, the height of the waves (amplitude) which indicates the relative voltage or power of each wave, the shape of the waves, and the patterns formed by groups of different waves. From this he can make assumptions about such disorders as epilepsy, brain tumors, damage from head injury or stroke, and encephalitis. The alpha machine is not usually attached to a print-out mechanism and therefore tends to indicate merely the presence and relative strength of a particular wave, rather than its specific characteristics. This, however, is all that is needed for most forms of alpha training.

The Brain Waves

Brain waves are measured and described in terms of their frequencies or cycles per second. They form a continuous spectrum all the way from zero cps (death) up to 60 or 70 cps (certain types of drug coma). They have been broken down into groups of frequencies, however, both for convenience in referring to them and because there seem to be peaks of voltage at various points along the continuum which may mark off somewhat different phenomenon. It has been suggested that each type of brain wave is associated with a distinctly different state of mind or mode of mental functioning. If this is true it is conceivable that training with mechanisms such as the current alpha machines will allow us to choose a desired state of consciousness at will with practice.

Alpha waves were both the first to be identified as well as one of the most basic brain wave phenomena. They tend to have the highest voltages (the greatest electrical power) of any of the brain waves, with a peak at about 10 to 12 cps. The alpha rhythm is generally identified as those frequencies from 8 through 13 cps. They are the dominant rhythm in a normal adult EEG record where the subject is relaxed, awake and his eyes closed. "Alpha blocking," or the sudden shutting off of alpha wave production by the brain, can be caused voluntarily by opening the eyes or performing a task requiring focused attention, such as mental arithmetic. It can result involuntarily from a sudden external stimulus, such as a loud noise. A lack of alpha waves under the conditions described above is sometimes a warning or danger signal, but there are many normal adults who do not produce alpha readily.

Delta waves are the slowest of the brain waves, appearing from time to time in sleep. They range from the first detectable activity up to 4 cps and peak in power between 1 and 2 cps. Slow waves are common in young children as a normal part of their development.

Theta waves, falling between 4 and 7 cps, are little understood but attracting more attention lately. Their appearance in the deepest meditation of some Zen masters may indicate that they have considerable importance to those interested in alpha training. Dr. Barbara Brown, Chief of Experimental Physiology at the Veterans Administration Hospital in Sepulveda, California, and one of the leading researchers in this field, has commented that theta appears to be related to "problem solving, sorting and filing of incoming data and retrieval of information already deposited in the brain's memory. Theta training," she feels, "may very well facilitate awareness, enhance memory and, in general, lead to a sensational increase in the efficiency with which the mind works," although this is still unproven.

Beta waves commonly include all waves faster than alpha —from 14 cps on up. Their voltage peak, or greatest strength, is about 20 to 25 cps. They appear in normal adults who are "alert" as opposed to relaxed. Being "in beta" has become the alpha machine salesman's jargon for that tense, irritable state which is unpleasant to experience and often unpleasant to be around. He is offering to sell you a machine which will teach you to "get into alpha" and thereby feel better, look better, and do better. This is probably a bit simplistic. It is more likely that beta has its legitimate functions, just as alpha does, and is the most effective state for many of the tasks we have to perform.

The four basic wave forms mentioned were recognized early and have been confirmed repeatedly in EEG research. More recent and still more questionable phenomena include kappa waves and gamma waves. Gamma waves have the same frequencies as alpha waves but much smaller voltages. The term gamma waves is sometimes used to refer to those very fast beta waves which have a voltage peak around 50 cps. These are also referred to simply as "very fast beta waves" (anything from 30 cps on up) and can be seen in adults who have taken quantities of certain drugs.

An individual's brain waves fluctuate a great deal from hour to hour and even from moment to moment. This depends on such factors as state of consciousness (sleep, resting, alert), the degree and type of emotional arousal (how good or bad you feel), the use of drugs and the presence of sickness or injury. There are not distinctly different patterns for every one of these states, however, and reading your brain waves is in no way comparable to reading your mind. In fact, one could probably get better clues about what you are thinking by looking at your face and your posture. Very few of these states could be identified from their EEG records alone. On the other hand, in spite of their diversity, each individual tends to have a rather distinct set of patterns. A skillful EEG technician could probably match up several of your EEG's taken at different times, even if they were mixed in with the records of a number of other people. Heredity seems to play a part in this, just as it does in determining our basic temperament. For example, identical twins, who share the same genetic struc-

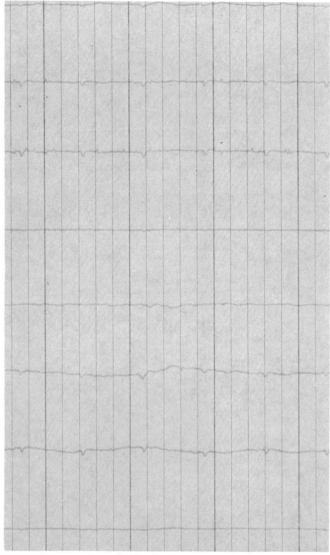

EEG pattern from a brain that has no electrical activity. The subject is legally dead but the heart continues to emit faint impulses that are recorded as small amplitude waves or blips. Each line represents an electrode attached to the head.

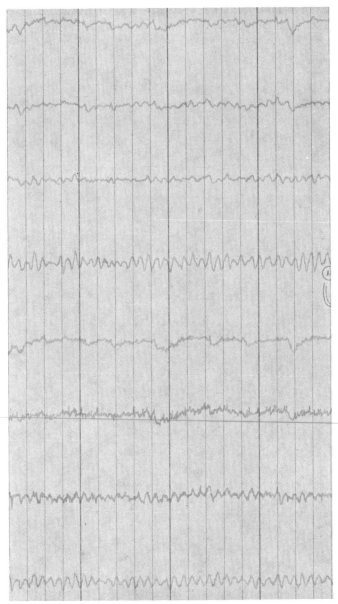

EEG pattern demonstrating predominantly alpha rhythm (8-13 cps).

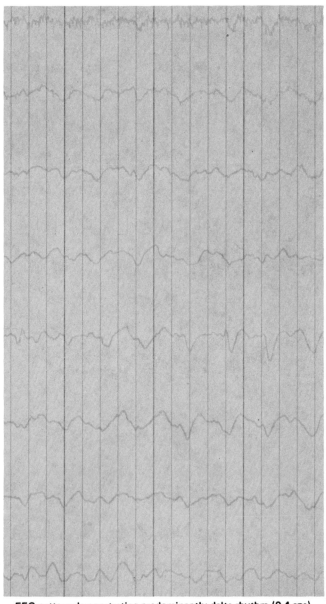

EEG pattern demonstrating predominantly delta rhythm (0-4 cps).

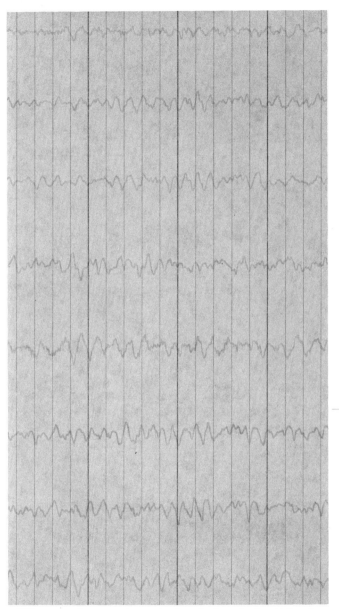

EEG pattern demonstrating predominantly theta rhythm (4-7 cps).

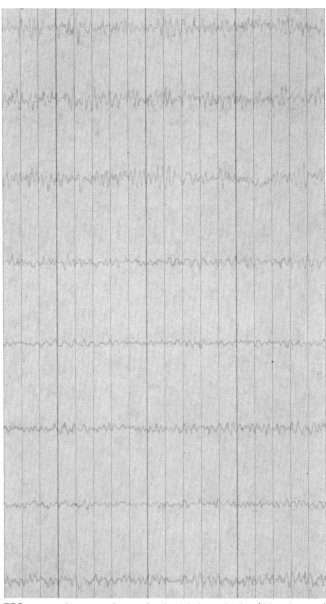

EEG pattern demonstrating predominantly beta rhythm (14 and up cps).

ture, have EEG records which are more similar to each other than to other members of their family. And the EEG abnormalities found in epileptics are sometimes also found in the records of their blood relations who do not have this disorder. To a certain degree then, brain wave patterns are passed along from one generation to the next.

Investigators have found that by placing electrodes at various points around the head different wave types are stronger in different areas and seem to originate primarily from these areas. Alpha waves are most easily read from the back of the head over the "visual cortex," that part of the brain which analyzes visual stimuli. It is especially interesting, therefore, that the waves are strongest when the eyes are shut and the waves can be blocked by concentrating intently on visual images. In fact, individuals who tend to use much visual imagery in their thinking seem to produce alpha less readily than those who think more abstractly. The faster waves (beta and gamma) seem to come from the forward parts of the brain, which are generally associated with reasoning and emotion. There has been some speculation that delta waves normally come from deep within the brain (the hypothalamus). They are also known to arise in the cortex around tumors and injuries to brain tissue and can be used to locate them. In spite of their having apparent sources in the brain of man, studies of other animals and of other parts of the body besides the brain show that "brain waves" seem to be a characteristic of any mass of nerve tissue. They probably represent the cumulative electrical fields from the activity of many separately functioning nerve cells. So far no one knows definitely whether brain waves actually originate at the point where they seem to be the strongest or not. It is also not known whether they represent thousands of cells working together at the same frequencies or whether they are the cumulative electrical effect of many diverse neural functions. The reason for stressing the ignorance of scientists in this area is to help you evaluate popular claims for brain waves. The nervous system is immensely complex and still not well understood. Anyone who claims to have exact knowledge about brain waves must be at least provisionally suspected of being a mystic, a charlatan or a fool.

What is Biofeedback?

Most alpha sets are sold for the simple purpose of learning to produce more alpha waves. This is really part of the more general process of biofeedback training. It refers to the fact that in the last few years scientists of the West have realized for the first time that many bodily processes thought to be fully automatic and involuntary could be brought under conscious control if the proper circumstances were created.

If you intend to strap some electrodes to your head and listen to the sounds of your brain in the hope of learning to increase your alpha you will be engaging in a form of biofeedback training. Regardless of whether your goal is wisdom, relief from anxiety, or a brain wave high your chances of success will be increased if you understand the process.

Learning might be divided for our purpose into two types, that which is passively recorded (book learning) and that knowledge which is developed through experimentation. The second type is much more pervasive. It is a part of all our behavior all through our life and for this reason we are much less aware of it. Unlike studying in school it is not something we do on well-defined occasions. It is the way we live. We have forgotten that we once learned how to walk or to swallow and breath alternately so we wouldn't choke. The tendency is to think of these things as automatic and occurring without thought, but if you could become aware that they once represented a real challenge (watch a young child) you are less likely to become discouraged if you do not produce alpha immediately and constantly just because you will it. It is understanding and not force of will which is the key.

One of the vital elements of such experimentation is feedback. That simply means knowing just how well you did each time you tried so that you can correct yourself next time. It is a more or less gradual process which requires repetition for success. The alpha machine provides feedback. That is all it does.

Any benefits you may get from increasing your alpha production will come entirely from yourself. The machine will only provide a missing link in the learning cycle. In this case the cycle has been called a *biofeedback loop* because you make an attempt to alter a biological process, the machine measures your success and reports it back to you so you can try to correct yourself and begin again. Around and around it goes until you are satisfied.

This seems to be a form of operant conditioning, which means learning to control your operations (behavior) by receiving constant rewards or punishments which guide you ever closer to your goal. In this case the rewards or punishments come entirely from you. You feel good if you are achieving what you set out to do and bad every time you don't. If you get too discouraged, for instance by expecting too much too soon, you may condition yourself to avoid the whole thing and give up trying.

Too much anxiety blocks learning which is why trying too hard is usually counterproductive. This is especially true of learning to produce alpha waves, since they *only* seem to emerge in relaxed states. If you tend to be an overanxious person it will probably be harder for you to learn to control your alpha. On the other hand, it does seem likely that there could be some benefits for you if you stick with it. This does not make any specific claims for alpha waves themselves, but the association of alpha with relaxation is one of the few relatively solid facts in this area. If you somehow do learn to produce alpha at will you will probably have learned to deal with your anxiety in the process. Even if none of the other claims are borne out this will still be one fact with a real potential to benefit you.

The Problem of Self-Awareness

There are some very real difficulties you are likely to encounter in trying to do this. In spite of the fact that this form of conditioning is automatic it is probably a gross oversimplification to look at yourself as just a bundle of conditioned reflexes.

Sitting still, being quiet, and maintaining a relaxed and open state of mind are some of the most difficult things humans can do. Animals have been taught to control brain waves and a number of other physiological processes but they probably don't have to deal with the same type of inner turmoil as human beings must.

Being really quiet can be irritating. It can be depressing. It can be frightening. There are things buried in each of us that we do not like to face. They take time and courage to accept and place into perspective, until finally, we can use them as valid parts of our personalities and not waste large portions of our energy *not knowing* about them. When we are not distracted by being busy with the world they have a tendency to bubble up like great psychic belches from that undigested portion of our psyche to cause emotional heartburn. Usually, instead of recognizing what is happening we prefer to say we are bored, become fidgety, and look around for something else to do. We return to being busy.

One of the basic reasons why the psychoanalyst sits behind the patient and says little (assuming he is not asleep, as depicted in so many cartoons) is to avoid distracting the patient's attention from himself, his inner self. Students of Zen recognize this phenomenon and, indeed, those who attempt any form of meditation must eventually come to deal with it somehow. That is probably why those who are experienced at some form of meditation do better with alpha machines right from the start. It is difficult and usually takes time. This is one reason why Zen and analysis involve years.

It is entirely conceivable that an alpha machine can be used in the same way, although this is just beginning to be explored. One of the basic functions of the Zen master and the therapist is to repeatedly point out to an individual in their charge when he is distracting himself from his supposed task: attention to himself. Patients frequently become angry with the therapist at this point. Your alpha machine will fulfill the same function to a certain extent. Don't be surprised if you become enraged at a machine which nags you for not doing what you set out to do. That's why you bought it.

This is not to suggest that an alpha machine is a valid substitute for psychotherapy. On the other hand, *if* you are able to listen to and deal with the disruptive voices from within yourself while you are learning to relax and produce alpha, a great deal of self-knowledge could quite possibly result. It will not come from the alpha, but from your struggle to find it. These same benefits could also come from just sitting quietly and really listening to yourself at regular intervals. It is just that most of us need some guidance in this process. Because of these very human difficulties it would not be surprising if many of the alpha machines which were purchased were not used for more than a few weeks at most. It is for the same reasons that approximately half of all the patients who come for psychotherapy leave within the first few sessions, despite their need.

There may be legitimate reasons for abandoning the alpha machine also. Not everyone seems to get the same benefits from the experience. Some individuals become relaxed and aware while others apparently just fall asleep. There are conflicting reports that, on the one hand, representatives of the hip drug culture do poorly at producing alpha, and on the other, that those with previous (sometimes drug) experiences with peak feelings are more likely to repeat them during brain wave training. Reports vary from ecstasy and states of enhanced creativity to just O.K. Apparently no one who has succeeded in producing alpha actively dislikes the experience, but it may do different things to different people. Undoubtedly one's expectations and general attitudes toward this type of experience, degree of suggestibility, and emotional style all play a role.

The Question of Danger

The issue has been raised about the possibility of actual danger from using alpha machines. Manufacturers and distributors tend to deny that there is any problem here. They point out that the machines do nothing to you, put nothing into your head, and you yourself respond only as you wish to when using one. Their only real cautionary note is against plugging accessory jacks into outside power sources because of the unpleasant possibility of electrocution. This restriction should be taken seriously. The manufacturers' position appears to be essentially reasonable. A few qualifications are worth noting, nonetheless.

Dr. Brown mentioned her concern in an article in *Los Angeles Times West*. They mainly have to do with the possibility that under certain conditions alpha machines may pick up signals which are not part of normal brain function. An unlucky individual may put a lot of time and effort into learning a pathological process or something which is not at all to his benefit, without realizing it. If electrodes are incorrectly placed so that muscle signals rather than alpha are picked up the individual will get the mistaken impression that he is increasing his alpha every time he activates those particular muscles. The machine only detects electrical activity and it is up to the user to distinguish between the different types of signals. In this case one might actually be conditioning himself to be more tense and may end up with a headache rather than the peaceful repose of alpha. Similarly, if the electrodes pick up heartbeats the alpha trainee would get his feeling of accomplishment by learning to speed up the rate of his heart but he would be unlikely to benefit from the experience.

Potentially more serious was the case reported by Dr. Brown of a woman who was learning to produce epileptic spikes (sudden violent electrical discharges from the brain which are associated with epileptic seizures) without being aware of it. It is conceivable that under these circumstances someone with a minor trace of epileptic-type activity could amplify it over time until fullblown seizures resulted. Fortunately, this type of problem seems quite a rare occurrence with the use of alpha machines.

There also remains the quite general questions regarding the effects of altering the normal activity of the brain. This is not as sinister as it might seem. It may be "normal" for some of us to be quite tense, but it is usually more healthy to alter this state. Alpha training may do little more than that. There has not been any accumulation of complaints regarding the relatively short-term training involved in most scientific experiments and, in fact, the experience has been almost uniformly pleasant for those involved. On the other hand, the long-term effects can only be known when large numbers of individuals practice alpha enhancement over a period of years. If you are intending to use a machine regularly it would be wise to keep yourself informed of any developments in this field.

Getting Off on Alpha

To get the most out of your alpha training you will have to strike a balance between being reasonable and cautious and being relaxed and open to the experience. The time and trouble of wiring yourself to most machines may make this difficult at first. It takes practice to place the electrodes properly and to learn how to adjust your machine. Especially at the beginning there will probably be days when your attention will be tied up in life problems and cannot be allowed to float freely. When you are starting out it will probably be better to abandon the attempt any time you feel you are definitely not in the mood. You cannot force alpha out of your brain with determination. It is a state you have to relax into. Once you have had the experience of some success with it, things will probably go a lot more smoothly during most training sessions. If you do have occasional states of jangled nerves afterwards you will then have a much better sense of how to deal with them without getting still more tense and discouraged in the attempt.

You should pick a comfortable place to sit or lie, at least at first. Later on you might want to see just how much stress you can subject yourself to and still maintain your alpha-cool, but at the outset keep it as simple as possible. Distractions should be at an absolute minimum. Dim lighting may help.

A common experience of neophytes is that they will start to produce alpha, the machines will signal them that this is so, and they will become preoccupied with their success. This has the disappointing effect of shutting off the alpha again. It may be necessary to go through this process a number of times before the feeling of accomplishment can be taken casually and not distract one.

The other side of the "self-awareness problem" is quite positive and encouraging. Individuals who increase their openness and become more relaxed, who learn to let their feelings and awareness flow more readily, commonly experience a tremendous surge of energy. This represents one type of peak experience many have reported. It is often accompanied by intense joy and a feeling of the freshness of life. When energy which was knotted up in the attempt to protect the psyche is released suddenly we often feel free and happy and can then use our abilities more effectively. If alpha training does that for you, you will probably think it was well worth the effort.

3

The Coming of Alpha

> ...most of what is presently happening that is new,
> provocative, and engaging in politics, education, the
> arts, social relations ... is the creation either of youth
> ... or of those who address themselves primarily to
> the young.

Theodore Roszak made the above statement in his book, *The Making of a Counter Culture*—and if Mr. Roszak is correct then the current alpha wave phenomenon clearly meets the "new criteria" for what qualifies things as "new, provocative and engaging." When new things appear on the horizon, we naturally expect that there will be some connection between our new phenomenon and this strange animal called *Youth*. It is not surprising, therefore, that the people who are first being drawn to and becoming involved with alpha are the young.

Some people would argue that this is the way things have always been. They would say that the past has also known youth movements that have resulted in major social changes.

But still there pervades a feeling of "Yes, but not quite like this, not just this way." As social scientists of a different era look back at us and the 1970s, it may be from a perspective that sees the greatest significance of our entire era as the strange manner with which our culture had come to deal with things new. It would be as if Wilbur and Orville Wright had made their historic flight at Kitty Hawk only to discover that no one over thirty had noticed they could fly.

If Sigmund Freud had just completed the manuscript *Civilization and Its Discontents*, the layman would probably learn of his teachings through the pages of the *Evergreen Review* and the *Berkeley Barb* long before *Time* hit the stands with its special report. The first schools to offer courses on his writings would be the free universities, long before it would be included in the course catalogues at UC Berkeley. (That is what happened with transactional analysis. That is what *IS* happening with alpha.) It would be hard to believe that the first throngs coming to Freud's doors would again be the upper middle-class Viennese women, wanting to know how they ticked. Instead people would come from the college campuses, wise in the ways of Synanon games, encounter, sensitivity, drugs and Zen. Probably cults would form and vague references to libido would appear in the lyrics of Dylan and Lennon. An irate father somewhere would write the *New York Times* wanting to know why laws weren't being passed against these new cults. (Some researchers have already expressed this very fear of measures being taken against the use of alpha.)

Possibly the only thought which immediately crystalizes is the fact that the 1970s are in a different world than Freud's. Scientists can no longer hide behind ethical arguments of professional autonomy. The world that is science cannot disassociate itself from the world that is social. Understanding today's technological breakthroughs requires an understanding of them that is not only scientific, but social—and it means knowing who needed the breakthrough in the first place, who flocks to it and why.

It was the fate of alpha to be discovered in the midst of a revolution. And almost immediately it appears that the forerunners of both alpha and the ongoing revolution are somehow bound up with each other. Some see alpha as a part of the revolution or even the logical conclusion of it. It has already been seen by some as the ultimate psychedelic, as well as the ultimate method of weight control and the possible replacement for aspirin. The study of alpha still qualifies for at least one more ultimate. For in fact, at least scientifically, alpha represents science's ultimate probe into the fundamental workings of the human mind—purely and scientifically what makes it work, what makes us work. If there is any truth to the old adage about necessity being the mother of invention, we then have the task of wondering just who it is among us that finds a need for answers to those kinds of questions; the evidence, at least to this date, seems to be telling us: It is the young.

Shopping for Identity at the Old Identity Store

Dr. Joseph Kamiya, a research psychologist with San Francisco's Langley Porter Neuropsychiatric Institute, is considered one of the foremost explorers in the domain of alpha waves. He began to be discussed in the media in the late 1960s. It is interesting that his writings on the mental processes had their greatest followers among the youth. This, after all, was not merely the generation of psychedelic, mind-bending drugs but also of sensitivity and encounter groups, Synanon, transcendental meditation, yoga, astrology, Hare Krishna and rock concerts.

If we really want to know how it was that we have spawned such a generation with such desperation, the current state of things would probably tell us that we really don't have to look very deeply for our answers. It all started very simply. Back in the early 1960s the demands and goals of the revolution seemed very simple and clearly defined. Simple folksingers sang simple tunes about peace and brotherhood. Even if one did not agree, he did not really have to bend his mind far to at least understand what was being talked about. An end to the war? O.K. Equality for blacks? Sounds logical. At least, back then, the battles between the emerging New Left and the old middle existed in terms that weren't too offensive to anyone. Sit-ins, demonstrations and voter registration drives were mild compared to the violence of the 70s.

Then

In part, our understanding of what is happening is clouded by the fact change is occurring so rapidly that it is difficult to recall where things were only ten years ago. Even then it was obvious that a very wide rift had opened between those of middle age and a very vocal and disenfranchised contingency of the young. Back then the optimists of the great middle were probably correct when they referred to dissidents as being only a very small minority.

Perhaps more crucial is the fact that aside from its numbers the very tone and core of what was considered dissidence was far different from what exists now. In 1961 there was little said about drugs, aside from marijuana. Existence of most of the hard core psychedelics was not even known, and later we will see that the drugs themselves had a very crucial role to play in moving this unique generation to the place where it is today.

There were no Weathermen in 1961. The SDS from which they split was still nonviolent, as was most of the movement of which SDS comprised only a part. In fact while critics today spend much time belaboring the radical's obsession with violence, the young of the last decade seemed to be obsessed almost 180° the other way. Billboard notices referred not to demonstrations, but to nonviolent demonstrations. The word *nonviolent* found its way into the names of many of the new organizations which were then flourishing. In 1961 it was groovy to say you were a pacifist. Even as recently as 1966, when radical whites still comprised over one-half of the civil rights movement, the biracial demonstrations of Martin Luther King preached the concept of nonviolence almost as if it, itself, were a religion. The demonstrators he led through Chicago's West Side did not leave from their South Side rallying point until they were given a firm grounding in the principles of nonviolence. This was something he stressed almost as much as he stressed the need for the demonstration in the first place. Classes were held. "If you can't keep cool, we don't need you," he said. And his marchers were instructed not to hit back even if they themselves were struck. This is how it was through much of the early 1960s when the crouch of a civil rights demonstrator being beaten seemed to fill the pages of newspapers across the nation.

In 1961, if one wanted to find the radicals, the logical place to look would have been the college campus. Theodore Roszak notes this as a very important point, for the clustering of thirty thousand bodies on university campuses "has served to crystallize the group identity of the young." Much of what was happening—even in the far away streets of Selma—seemed to have its grounding and do its recruiting somewhere at the university.

It was an era where being a *beatnik* still seemed to have a lot to do with being an intellectual. In fact reading the right poetry and novels and listening to the right kind of jazz were the very factors which would often categorize one as a *beatnik*.

Perhaps the real essence of how things differed then and now is simply in the very mood, the very way in which people talked to each other. A drop-out cab driver (formerly a government employee), whose birthdate strategically allowed him to pass through both the beat and hip eras while in his mid-twenties, says:

> You can see a real difference simply looking at the parties. Back then everybody'd get stoned and sit around talking to each other. Now that's archaic. Music's too loud anyway. About all you can do is smile at each other and gyrate...
> I think a lot of the difference is basically because

the whole thing was still new then. We were excited with what we were doing. I'm sure drugs have contributed to the change too. And when people do talk now that's what most of the conversation is about. Then it was politics. Now if you're cool, you're apolitical.

Now

The apoliticalism among the young cited by the cab driver has grown to such proportions that it seems to have hit its zenith. The trend now is basically away from the system. Those who have become part of the "Back-to-the-Earth" movement and members of communes are probably leading an existence as far removed from the system as is possible while still residing within the borders of the United States. Obviously not everyone under thirty has taken to this extreme. But many of those who have stayed behind seem to be finding life-styles further and further removed from what is considered as the mainstream of society. It is almost as if the young have unilaterally decided that from now on they are going to do for themselves what society has refused to do.

In the city of San Francisco there are free clinics dispensing medical services the government does not provide. There are free universities teaching subjects the state-funded schools refuse to teach. In the San Francisco Bay area there are several full-time switchboards run by the young which do nothing else but direct people to the services they are seeking.

For many of the young, the list of society's offerings which they have rejected includes not only its affluence, values and language, but even its food. For some of those persons taken up in the trend toward organics, a pound of supermarket "enriched" flour is a pound of poison. Organizations such as the Food Conspiracy have sprung up in which young people take care of their own food distribution, thus essentially bypassing the need for stores entirely.

And what all of this adds up to is quite obvious: There *is* a counterculture, a society within a society. In many ways it would be difficult to conjure up a rift that is more complete.

Searching for One's Head

If the science of psychology has something to do with "looking inward" then the beginnings of the current inward trend occurred in the mid1950s. This sudden emergence occurred, significantly, not merely on the college campus but in the mind of the general public as well. In 1957 an article in *Life* magazine noted that one movie out of every ten was either about a psychiatrist or else included one. At that time the public demand for mental service was exploding at such a rate that it was estimated the need for practicing psychologists would double in just a few years.

In the beginning the trend to look inward was a phenomenon that included not just the young but everybody. But it did not remain that way.

The generation which is now said to have dropped out became involved with psychology from both ends, as doctors and as patients. Enrollment began to swell in university departments of social science as well as in the number of names on the waiting list to see the campus psychiatrists in the health centers. In the early stages, the brand of psychology with which the young had begun to involve themselves was a psychology of a very traditional nature. It became more or less Freudian, depending on which university the student happened to be attending.

We have already seen that those things which become the concern of the young do not remain static for long. It was the same with psychology. As the first major overhauls began in psychological methodology it was the generation over thirty which began to drop out; it was the young who became attracted in overwhelming numbers.

The real shift began in the mid1960s as the spread of sensitivity groups began, initially, on the college campuses. This sensitivity methodology, which was picked up quite rapidly, rests on a very simple premise: Modern life allows for a very small degree of feeling. When we do have emotions our social impulse is not to express but, rather, to repress them.

The particular focus of any one sensitivity group may vary considerably from the next. The phenomenon has been around long enough for a wide variety of schools of thought to develop, and, consequently, varied methods begin to make this appearance. There are some groups which shun entirely the idea of verbal communication. One San Francisco group, meeting for the first time, began its sesssion with an hour and a half of rubbing backs, after which the leader asked, "Shall we all go home with this wonderful high? Or should we talk and ruin it?" The consensus was to go home with the "wonderful high."

To some this may have the sound of an incredible affectation (one member of that group just mentioned expressed this very feeling). But if it is an affectation it is at least an affectation with a theory behind it. Verbal communication, many sensitivity theorists would argue, is where all our defenses are at. As soon as talk begins, the defenses crop up.

Not all sensitivity groups are totally nonverbal. For it is also believed that the verbal expression of feelings is also something which society has trained us not to do. At many groups, the central focus resides simply in attempting to open up a level of communication in which its members can address each other in terms of their true feelings.

The spread of sensitivity groups has been so vast that they are now included in the curricula of some of the more experimental high schools. The same holds true for several universities which require this course as part of the four-year college education.

The distinction between encounter groups and sensitivity groups becomes somewhat foggy. In general it could be said that the encounter groups tend to rely more on verbal communication and are more open-ended in terms of their goals. Some groups encompass the sensitivity concept of getting in touch with feelings. But, to many, encounter is simply a vehicle by which to meet other people without the painful small talk that normally precedes most social relations. Some people join the groups to work out particular problems; still others find it just a good time. For whatever reasons they join the groups the underlying theme is to become involved with each other. The role of the group leader, if there is one, is to direct the group members toward each other. His role is also to maintain a watch over the prevailing ground rules, assuring that things do not go too far beyond the relevant.

In encounter the emphasis is on the here and now; whatever one is feeling at the moment becomes relevant. One is encouraged to take the risk of expressing that feeling rather than supressing it. If a male in the group is attracted to a female, he is encouraged to say so (rather than to sit and think about it). Frequently a group leader will begin to break down peoples' defenses by simply asking the members of the group to state to whom they are attracted. Many encounter members seem to find this quite a relief from the usual roundabout ways people normally get together.

At encounter, people have the opportunity to work directly on their problems. A shy male student from the University of California at Berkeley told his fellow group members that he could not escape from his fear of people because he always felt as if he were below everybody. Someone in the group suggested that it might help if he stood up and gave everybody orders; this he did for thirty minutes.

As the interest in encounter groups has spread so has their scope. Recently very specialized groups have sprung up which deal with very specific problems in human relations: male-female encounter, black-white encounter, gay encounter, women's lib encounter to name a few.

Another form of encounter already being considered for the future is alpha encounter. Vague references have been made to this concept by several users of the alpha machines. It basically amounts to exploring how people in similar alpha states may relate to each other. And it would seem only natural that alpha and the encounter phenomenon should have a common meeting ground, for it has already been observed that it is predominantly the same people who are attracted to both.

A common link between sensitivity and encounter group is the assumption that the barriers which people place between each other are best done away with in a gentle, nonhostile atmosphere in which every member of the group has an equal responsibility to break down his own defenses. But there is another form of encounter which takes an approach that is almost the direct opposite—that of Synanon.

Synanon attempts to break through a person's defenses by bulldozing right past them. When attention focuses on a certain group member it would probably appear to an outsider as if everyone else in the group had simultaneously decided to attack him. Often the attacks are not gentle; many persons have criticized the Synanon approach on the basis that it becomes very difficult for one to let down his defenses when he perpetually finds himself in the state of being attacked.

However, a great many Synanon participants are people who are hard-core users of drugs, and it is argued that these are people who have become so lost in their defenses that there is simply no other way of breaking through.

Nondrug users also attend Synanon sessions. Many of them eventually drop out, finding that its hard-core approach is more than they care to deal with. One former member, a doctor who now attends an encounter group, says:

> What scared me so much at Synanon was that I had become so good at it. I was mostly among hard-core drug users, and at least in them I could see some justification for the pent up hostilities they were releasing; but to find the feelings in myself was frightening.

No matter what brand of the new psychology we add to our list—whether it be, for example, primal therapy or psychodrama—we would find that, by and large, its adherents are young people. This is a common bond which presently seems more critical than the very ideology from which these offshoots of "head science" have grown. If we still must ask why it is that the young are going there, we have only to look at the very thing they do when they arrive—an answer which almost seems obvious—they are looking into their heads and into the heads of others. When we extend the question to, "Yes, but why do they do THIS?" the question becomes virtually absurd. It is what men have always done and, perhaps, a better question might be, "Whatever happened to the curiosity of the old?"

Expanding One's Head Once One Has Found It

Drugs exist. This bare, unadorned fact is of particular concern to us because people invented drugs, and people take drugs. What drugs represent is yet another means of exploring the murky, unknown phenomenon that men refer to as minds.

The human mind, basically, is a machine—the second known to mankind (the first being his body). It is the machine we know least about. A researcher in the science of neurophysiology once stated that perhaps it says something about man that he came to understand the workings of his rear end before his mind.

Even the most current findings tell us only what minds do, not how they do it, why they do it and how those factors can be controlled.

In dealing as we have been with the social dynamics of just what it is that impels the younger generation toward these inner excursions of the mind, the presence of drugs creates a problem. This problem is similar to those encountered by people trying to solve the chronology of chickens and eggs. What produces what? Has the phenomenon of drugs created interest in the mind, leading to an upsurge in the "new psychology?" Or has the new psychology.... Some of those people interviewed in the process of collecting data for this book have expressed both preferences. If a hasty conclusion were to be drawn, it would be that neither the chicken nor the egg came first because they both did.

We are, however, somewhat better versed in the genesis of contemporary chickens as we know, categorically, that eggs have preceded every one of them. Alpha is the chicken of which drugs and the new psychology were eggs, laid, of course, by a chicken named social unrest and alienation.

What drugs and the new psychology have done, then, for the cause of alpha research has been to bring to it an energetic following. With drugs in particular there are two added factors which have brought about this union. Firstly, there has been the discovery that people undergoing alpha training have been known to experience states of euphoria and well-being, which resemble the experiences of many of the users of psychedelics. And however this speaks for the case of alpha it cannot be denied that some of the new devotees are around for kicks. As euphoria and well-being are two well-known states of the human consciousness (desirable ones at that) there is nothing unscientific or irrelevant in the study of their physiological dynamics.

The second factor, a bit more philosophical, deals with the often stated reports of drug users that they return from their highs with an openness to new things which they did not previously possess.

A young woman in San Francisco, involved in teaching the use of the alpha machine, directly correlates her involvement with alpha to her previous experience with drugs:

> They made me aware that there are such things as states of consciousness in which people can achieve a calmness of mind and body. And naturally I am interested in ways in which these things can be controlled.

Ironically, the very source which brings popular backing to the study of alpha may also end up as one of its detriments. For if further research does reveal easily controlled, drug-like experiences, it is only likely that alpha will come to be used for those purposes. At that point it is certain to be watched very carefully by the same people who scrutinized LSD closely enough to pass a law against it. For, like alpha, LSD began as a scientific discovery with exciting possibilities. It has been discovered in 1938. That was long before Timothy Leary had inspired a great deal of psychological research. This was due largely to the belief that it brought on a state of mind resembling that of many psychoses (something now disputed). But then came Leary, a revolution and a law. The law really had very little effect on the street usage of the drug, while it has almost entirely stifled the scientific exploration. As a consequence, those who use it are left the alternatives of proceeding in ignorance or not proceeding at all.

The Search for God

"If God did not exist, it would be necessary to invent him." When Voltaire made that statement it is improbable that he foresaw a time when his thesis would ever come to an empirical test. However, it seems that this is precisely what is happening. Among the many factors which separate this generation from others is the fact that it is probably the first generation for many centuries that has grown up without a god.

In rejecting almost the total spectrum of what society has handed down, the traditional faiths have gone by the same wayside as has, say, the forty-hour week. The younger generation has had to face the dilemma of doing without a faith altogether, or finding a replacement.

Again we are forced to flash back to sometime before the Hare Krishna days to recall that as it all started in the late 1950s and early 1960s, the avant garde of the new generation was largely agnostic—just as were most of their emerging literary heroes and the then-popular philosophy of existentialism. There was, of course, a great deal of interest in religion, but it was the Eastern religions, along with the Eastern philosophy. Interest in these areas probably has not really diminished in the past decade. But there has been a great, almost unaccountable, expansion into areas which were then unheard of.

The recent birth of the youth movement, barely ten years old, is wrought with ironies. One of these ironies was perfectly stated by a professor who noted the incredible incongruity of the Berkeley campus, a campus generally conceded to be the intellectual frontrunner of the nation. And yet it is that campus in which there exists a student body deeply grounded in supernatural beliefs that smack of the Dark Ages.

On Telegraph Avenue in Berkeley, when people meet, the question, "What's your sign?" is almost a virtual certainty. The sudden boon back to the beliefs of old times includes not only astrology but also tarot cards, palmistry, I Ching and black magic. In Berkeley some student baby-sitters ask the sign of a child before they agree to sit. Even more startling is the fact that witchcraft covens now exist in many major U.S. cities.

Offering an explanation, an article in *Newsweek* on the spread of the occult says, "...at stake for those who become deeply involved with the occult... [is a reflection of] the same search for an emotional anchor that underlies many young people's drift towards drugs."

In a sense it appears as if there is a reemergence of the same trend away from rationality which inspired the Dadaist art movement of the 1920s after the close of World War I.

Protestant theologian Harvey Cox, in *Senior Scholastic*, states that the "...modern society ignores the non-rational dimensions of existence. The absurd, the inspiring, the uncanny, the awesome, the terrifying, the ecstatic—none of these fits into a production- and efficiency-oriented society."

The offering of Mr. Cox seems to square with many of the feelings expressed by the young themselves. In a response to an editorial in *Time* magazine, a nineteen-year-old girl wrote about her disenchantment with the shift from pacificism:

> What are we supposed to do with our lives? How do we go about solving the complex problems of our world? "Work with the system," we hear. "You are sound and strong."
> There comes a time when pure frustration breaks out and is ugly. You throw a bottle and it feels good. You say "f---" and it feels good. If you can't change it, blow it up. It becomes a very personal and illogical thing.

Another student, quoted in *Senior Scholastic* magazine states, "I'd sooner feel that my future was being shaped by the stars or by the turn of the cards. These would represent powers more concerned about me than would either my draft board or the Pentagon."

Another says, "...Why use the I Ching in a world where you have the IBM 360 computer? The answer is easy. You can't understand the 360 and you don't have much control over it. The I Ching says that there are powers that are more powerful than the 360—powers *you* can use to control your life."

Astrology and occult, of course, have both known brief surges of popularity since their birth long ago. But, as the same magazine notes, "Never before in history has a single society taken up such a wide range of religious and near-religious systems at once."

As to where it all started, we can look for an answer in Jacob Needleman's book, *The New Religions.* Mr. Needleman points the finger squarely at the state of California. This is where the coffeehouses, drugs and the warfare of generations began. Mr. Needleman finds that it is the natural birthplace for the new, unusual or downright weird. "This aspect of California is not, of course, limited to the religious. It is true of politics, food habits, sexual behavior, clothing, education, medical practices—probably every outré or extreme aspect of human behavior is well-housed here." Mr. Needleman concludes, "Something is struggling to be born here amid all the obvious absurdity and grotesquery."

It is in California, especially, where the interest in the Eastern faith has continued to prosper among the young. Looking further into this faith, we begin to find curious elements which seem to say a great deal about where this generation has gone and where it might go from here.

Mr. Needleman finds that a major difference between the Judeo-Christian and Asian teachings lies in how each appeals to the worshipper's question of "What's in it for me?" The Judeo-Christian reward, he says, is happiness, while in Asian teachings it is the release from suffering.

Here is where the pieces begin to fit together in a manner which is almost uncanny. Such terms as "release from suffering" coincide not only with the experience of the Buddhist Zen masters, but also sound very much like current reports of a drug experience. Another area where the same experiences might apply is in the realm of alpha.

Alpha seems to bring together widely divergent fields in strange sorts of ways. Science and religion, for example, long seemed to journey along their paths by going in almost opposite directions. One almost had to deny the other. The Zen masters' claims of inner control were things science once branded as impossible, and yet this feat has clearly been demonstrated as fact. And as alpha subjects have reported Zen-like states through the use of alpha wave control, it is also a curious finding, noted by students of alpha, that the Zen masters who have submitted themselves to research seem to generate higher pulses of alpha waves almost naturally. This seems to say that a phenomenon regarded by the West as religious ritualism does have a scientific basis after all. It is a finding that is shattering in itself; whatever else alpha research may lead to promises to be equally shattering as well.

* * *

Alpha is a machine, but a machine which holds a promise of giving to man a greater control and understanding of the other machine—namely ourselves. And in a sense it almost sounds like the dawning of science fiction writer Arthur C. Clarke's prophesy in *Profiles of the Future* that one day man and machine will be bound together into a single being.

4

A Matter Of Life and Death

A British scientist studying the health of bereaved families finds that physical complaints often take precedence over spiritual problems during the period of mourning. Three times as many London widows contact their physicians with physical symptoms as see their clergyman in the six months after their husbands die. The problem for older widowers is even more serious. After losing their wives they suddenly show a 50 percent jump in heart disease as compared with married men of the same age. He concludes that one can indeed die of a broken heart.

*   *   *

A similar scientific investigation finds that in the year after the death of a family member there is seven times more likelihood that one of the surviving members will die than in a comparable non-bereaved family.

An anthropologist reports that voodoo death can occur. After a tribe member feels that he has been cursed or has broken an important taboo he can die rapidly and for no apparent physical reason.

These accounts are currently interpreted by the scientific community as evidence that our feelings can influence our health to such an extent that they can even kill us. But for years reports of mysterious deaths were disregarded by laboratory investigators because they were inexplicable. One cannot will his heart to stop, it was pointed out, and anyone who doubted it was invited to try. Experts on the problem of suicide note how often attempts to kill oneself fail. Those who truly wish to die find they must give up wishing and put a great deal of planning and effort into the conventional methods for ending life. We don't die easily.

All this is somehow reassuring. For although science has been proclaiming for years that *mind* and *body* are not separate entities but different perspectives on the same basic processes, most of us have continued with the same old habits of thought. We recognize that our thoughts are often capricious, extreme and irresponsible. It is reassuring to think of physiology as the real substance of life which continues with business as usual no matter what is in our unpredictable heads. The gap between the two is being continually narrowed, however, challenged by the accumulating evidence in three related areas.

Clinical research into psychosomatic disease, for one, has a growing pool of data which indicates the significant role played by emotional factors in psychosomatic illnesses. Psychosomatic diseases, as distinguished from hypochondriacal complaints, are real diseases which can cause suffering and even death. Some types of high blood pressure, ulcers and asthma are commonly named examples. General stress, habitual anxiety or anger have long been considered to play a role in their onset. Lately, however, it is beginning to appear that even infectious diseases are affected in important ways by our emotional states. Although the mechanisms are not yet known, situations producing feelings of helplessness and frustration may make us more susceptible to germs and virus.

A second area is the careful documentation of unexplained deaths, some of which were cited at the beginning of this chapter, which confirms folk tales and physicians' anecdotes. Once this information was gathered by professional researchers the scientist was in the position of either having to believe that a voodoo curse can indeed kill, or that the state of mind of an individual who believes he has been cursed was sufficient to somehow disrupt the involuntary processes which support life in our bodies. The consensus seems to be that these processes can somehow be altered by feelings under certain circumstances. This is now being demonstrated in the laboratory. When wild Norway rats are placed in the proper experimental situation they appear to die in response to feelings of hopelessness.

The third area is the very recent unfolding of biofeedback training, of which alpha training is one small part. It turns out that we may, after all, be able to stop our hearts under the proper conditions.

There is reason to believe that we may someday reap great benefits by learning to accept responsibility for the regulation of our vital processes.

At this time biofeedback training offers the tantalizing possibility of gaining a new dimension of flexibility and control over our bodies. We may be able to be much more effective in dealing with pain and various physical and emotional handicaps. We may be able to push disease and death back a full step from where they now hem us in. There is the chance that we may be able to get more from our living than ever before. This is the strike which has caused a goldrush of hundreds of researchers to the biofeedback claims. It is little wonder.

After that inflammatory introduction a word of caution is in order. The preceding do seem like legitimate possibilities at this time and well worth serious investigation. But to the scientist a possibility is just that and no more. He recognizes the deeply human need to substitute what we wish for what really is. When he hears of breakthroughs which are dramatic and revolutionary he is doubly skeptical and cautious. We would do well to follow his example. On the other hand, once one recognizes that there can be no promises about the future then there is no reason not to be excited about what may be a whole new era of human discovery. Your taxes and contributions subsidize most of this work. You have paid your admission and may as well enjoy the show.

One of the primary targets for pioneering biofeedback researchers has been the circulatory system. This is at least partly due to the fact that circulatory disorders such as heart attack and stroke are major causes of disability and death in modern man. Control of blood pressure can have a significant effect upon these diseases as well as a number of related disorders. A sampling of recent research will give some idea of how far we have come in this direction. Many of the findings presented have to do with animal experiments. Preliminary work in any new area is usually done with animals, both for safety and convenience, before using human subjects.

A group of rats was rewarded every time they constricted the blood vessels in their tails (an easy place to measure the rate of blood flow in a rat) while another group was rewarded for dilating these vessels. Both groups learned to exercise reliable control over this function which had long been supposed to be completely involuntary. A potentially useful side effect discovered at this time was that body temperature could also be changed by this procedure. A similar experiment with college students (using the finger this time for measurement) showed that human subjects could also learn to control the size of their blood vessels when properly trained.

The small beginnings in this area have a potential for expanding importance which has captured the imagination of many an investigator. Cancer cells thrive and expand by drawing nourishment from the very organism they destroy. The same blood vessels which bring food and oxygen to healthy cells also feed the disease process. It has been hypothesized, however, that with enough selective control over blood flow, it would be possible to starve and kill tumors without surgery, harmful radiation or powerful drugs. Most current treatments which are strong enough to kill cancer cells will also damage healthy tissue or create unpleasant side effects. It may be possible someday to teach the body itself to reject a rampaging cancerous growth by closing down the feeding arteries and squeezing off its blood supply.

Several studies have demonstrated that rats can be taught to increase or decrease their heart rates as much as 20 percent. The changed rates at which their hearts beat were retained for as much as three months without further training. A very interesting discovery in conjunction with one of these studies indicated that rats which has been taught to increase their heart rates had difficulty learning to master certain tasks in later experiments while those which had been taught to slow their heart rates learned well afterwards. The finding suggests that altering heart rate may change one's emotional response to certain new situations and influence the ability to learn. Jumping ahead of the research for just a moment we might guess that modern man is not only straining his physical and emotional health by keeping himself in a state of rapid-pulsed tension but he also might be limiting his intellectual ability to deal with new situations.

Quite successful results were obtained in attempts to teach rats to raise and lower their blood pressure an average of 20 percent. This was accomplished selectively, without any change in heart rate or body temperature, suggesting that it may be possible to alter specific bodily processes through biofeedback training, in some cases without affecting related systems. This seems to be an advantage over many of the medical treatments now available. Human subjects have also been taught to control blood pressure through biofeedback and have achieved significant results within a single session.

The circulatory system is not the only function under consideration. Most of us tend to respond to all sorts of different life pressures with the same bodily symptoms, over and over through most or all of our lives. Some of us react to stress with skin problems, others with circulatory difficulties or with stomach trouble, intestinal reactions, headaches, loss of energy, etc. They are not adaptive reactions. That is, they do not help to solve the difficulties which put pressure on us, they only make things worse by making us sick also. (The sicknesses sometimes give us an excuse to withdraw from our problems, but that seldom solves anything.) It is not clear whether we somehow learned these reactions as children or if they represent some inborn tendency to respond in a particular biological way. But we do not need them and biofeedback may help us to modify them.

For example, rats have now been trained to both increase and decrease the contractions of the large intestine. This may hold much promise for sufferers of colitis. Irritability of the colon in humans can lead to diarrhea, weight loss, rectal bleeding, and, in some cases, even death. In spite of the difficulties modern medicine has had controlling this disorder there are indications that direct control may be possible in humans. Mastery of urethral and intestinal functions has already been claimed by some Yoga experts of the East. There are reports that Yoga masters have learned to relax their sphincters to such an extent that they can reverse the normal direction of flow and can suck up water into the bowel or bladder through the anus or penis.

Two additional animal studies are of interest because they demonstrate the remarkable extent to which control is potentially possible with biofeedback techniques. Two groups of rats were given opposite tasks. One was rewarded for increasing the rate of urine formation and one was rewarded for decreasing the rate. Each group learned to alter the rate of urine formation in the direction for which it was rewarded. Similar results were obtained in an experiment rewarding increased and decreased production of saliva in dogs. This was not accomplished by the classic Pavlovian method which starts by putting food before a hungry dog, but rather using a feedback loop to train the salivary gland directly.

The new methods are not confined to health issues Reading problems have also been treated through biofeedback techniques. One factor which significantly reduces reading speed is subvocalization. Even when reading silently and to ourselves many of us continue to "pronounce" words as we go. Although no sound or movement may be apparent to an observer, electronic measurement of muscle potentials in the throat show that the words are being mouthed silently. The habit is thought to originate from the exercise of reading aloud in class during the primary grades and later slows the movement of the eyes down to the slower rate at which we speak. This habit has been successfully eliminated by giving the reader feedback on the amount of movement in his throat while reading so he could discontinue it. An annoying noise sounds every time his throat muscles become active, while relaxing them will allow him to read in peace and quiet. Progress was quite rapid and reading speed improved noticeably.

Learning and behavior problems in disturbed children may also respond to biofeedback training. Miss Angie Nall, the Director of the Angie Nall School in Beaumont, Texas, works with children of average or above average intelligence who nonetheless have difficulty learning. Since bright, hyperactive children with learning difficulties are often suspected of having some brain damage, she routinely has EEGs given to her children upon admission. An examination of these records showed a relationship between an inability to concentrate on school work and the lack of a clear alpha pattern. In an attempt to remedy this seeming defect she gave alpha training to a group of these children for just half an hour a week for one month.

The results convinced her that alpha training could be helpful to these children. A particularly hyperactive boy showed dramatic improvement, as did another child with a stuttering problem. She is continuing the experiment at her school and also hopes that alpha training will offer at least a partial substitute for the tranquilizers and amphetamines which are usually given to such children to calm them and allow them to focus their attention.

Relaxation training may prove to be one of the areas where feedback is most effective and valuable. Muscle tension produces electrical signals which are even stronger and clearer than brain waves and the same type of machine can easily be modified so it will report either one, depending upon how the electrodes are placed. We are fortunate that muscle tension is now so easy to detect. Large numbers of modern man's complaints are primarily diseases of self-activation, another way of saying that we keep ourselves geared up for catastrophes which never come. Or we are too ready for the problems which do occur and are therefore too tense to deal with them effectively.

Muscle tension is work and it burns energy. If the tension is unnecessary then that is so much vital energy wasted. We all know the sensation of having to spend time in a boring, irritating or frightening situation and even if we did nothing but sit there, we leave more exhausted than if we had been working strenuously in more pleasant circumstances. That same energy could have been saved for physical, emotional or intellectual productivity if we had been able to relax in that situation.

One of the problems with relaxing, however, is in regard to knowing when we are tense. We tend to grow accustomed to stimuli which are constant, such as bad smells or loud noises, to accommodate ourselves to them, and to stop perceiving them. Individuals who are habitually tense are usually less aware of this than those around them who can see how they sit, stand and move. Urge someone like this to relax and he is likely to reply with irritation, "I am relaxed!" That is why, although there are some excellent methods for teaching relaxation and many individuals would benefit greatly from such training in terms of comfort and health, they are seldom prescribed as treatments. To learn to relax at will requires that one become sensitively attuned to when and where he is tense, an awareness which most of us screen out to various degrees. We need feedback to make real progress and until now this meant training with a professional or highly experienced observer.

The feedback machines seem likely to fill this gap. You can take one home with you after little or no training and practice as much as you want. Properly applied they can be more sensitive than the most expert human observer. Some individuals will probably still need to be supervised periodically by a relaxation therapist, but the number of individuals such an expert could treat should be greatly increased and the cost of treatment should go down significantly.

Relaxation training can be a valuable aid or even replacement for some types of psychotherapy. Some treatments already capitalize on the fact that you cannot be relaxed and anxious at the same time. Phobias (irrational fears), impotence and frigidity, and some learning blocks are examples of disorders of anxiety and tension which should yield to relaxation.

Generalized relaxation may be sufficient to alleviate many of these problems. This might be achieved for many as a simple by-product of alpha training. The link between heightened production of alpha waves and relaxation has been consistently reported by subjects in alpha training experiments. There is no scientific confirmation yet, however, as to whether this is an effective technique for the treatment of tension disorders.

For those who need the most direct relief in the shortest possible time and cannot afford the luxury of experimenting with the results of brain wave training another method is available. The *frontalis*, a muscle between the eyebrows, has been found to be a good indicator of the general level of muscular tension throughout the body. When it is relaxed you tend to be relaxed. When it is tense your forehead wrinkles in the well-known expression of worry. Attaching electrodes to this spot gives useful feedback concerning the success of one's attempts to unwind.

Victims of tension disorders such as vascular hypertension and chronic colitis have been found to show a marked inability to relax. They have been successfully trained to do so however, and after such instruction have been able to relax more fully, on the average, than an untrained group of normal subjects.

Tension and pain also form a destructive cycle. The body instinctively tenses in response to pain. Increased tension seems to heighten pain again, while also interfering with healing of some injuries which require rest. A group of patients with injury to the *trapezius* (a back and neck muscle which supports the head and raises the shoulders) were given relaxation training along with some healthy subjects. One group was given only the feedback they could get themselves from the sensation in their own muscles. Another group was hooked up to a biofeedback apparatus which reported back the myoelectric activity (muscle potentials). Feedback from the machine made for a significant improvement in all those who received it and although the injured group initially had much more difficulty relaxing, they were able to reach the same level of relaxation as the healthy subjects in just one training session in this experiment. This type of progress is extremely encouraging.

Also successful has been a two-barrelled biofeedback attack on insomnia. Sufferers from sleeplessness were first attached to machines which read and reported back on their muscle tension. This information allowed them to rapidly learn to relax their bodies when they wished it. Then they had electrodes from an EEG attached to their scalps and were signaled whenever they produced more of the slow brain waves which are associated with falling asleep. Individuals who had once taken as long as four hours to get to sleep were soon dropping off twice in a single 20-minute training session.

The United States Navy, among others, is understandably interested in the value of alpha states and relaxation. Psychologists are investigating to find out whether or not a person deprived of sleep could return himself to a state of alertness and effectiveness by putting himself into an alpha state for a period of time. If this were so then soldiers who mastered the technique would give their units a decided edge in combat or emergency situations. When the enemy began to drop from fatigue the biofeedback trained man could rest rapidly in alpha and then return to duty. Some preliminary work suggests that alpha states may be helpful in this way. Of course, it seems likely that every major industrialized nation is now or soon will be involved in the same type of research. A large volume of brain wave research is already being published behind the iron curtain, and this, like our own published research, represents only the unclassified work being done. We can only guess at the types of secret research being done here and in other countries.

Headaches also appear to be yielding to a multipronged approach. Although they have many causes the common varieties are generally divided into two groups: tension headaches and migraines. Tension headaches have responded quite rapidly in some instances to relaxation training. Migraines, which achieve their painful effect from the throbbing of blood vessels in the head, appear to be relieved somewhat by general relaxation, and even more so by relaxation in combination with feedback trained control of blood pressure or blood vessel constriction.

These everyday illnesses have led Americans to consume millions of pills yearly, to spend hours and days in suffering, and to feel trapped and helpless within their own bodies. If an experience as basic as this could be altered it seems likely to affect the way in which we think of ourselves and our functioning and will have repercussions throughout our society. The manufacturers of patent remedies and nonprescription drugs may not like it, but Americans may come to think of much sickness as a sign indicating they are having difficulty dealing with some aspect of their lives. The answer then would not necessarily be to pop a pill to relieve the symptoms, but to find out how to handle stresses more effectively. If one does not know how to dance he gets someone to teach him. If he has headaches because he doesn't know how to relax the same approach may be fruitful.

This puts more of the responsibility on the patient himself. Instead of taking himself to a druggist or doctor, as he brings a broken-down car to a mechanic, and saying "fix me," he might now say "teach me." The advantages are numerous. Physicians have recognized for some time that a major portion of patient complaints have some emotional basis. Recognizing this they often give advice about living (which is just as often disregarded) with their prescriptions. The prescription is mandatory, however, since the average American feels nothing has been done for him unless he receives a pill or an injection. As he comes to recognize the powerful effect his emotions have on his body he has a better chance to learn to get well and to stay well.

Physicians, too, will benefit. Less time will be tied up in repeatedly treating the recurrent symptoms of the same lingering illnesses and more could be devoted to medical emergencies. Instead of sending a patient home with medication, he might often leave with a specialized biofeedback training device and some instructions. After mastering the necessary techniques he should be able to deal with the problem on his own the next time it arises.

Tranquilizers and pain remedies are probably the most popular medications in America. In spite of the known side effects and dangers associated with many of them they are carried into some homes by the bushel full. These are usually intended to treat just those discomforts which may also be most accessible to biofeedback control. If the feedback method proves successful the advantages are likely to be considerable. Unpleasant reactions to drugs, the danger of addiction and considerable expense might all be done away with.

The prospects for preventive medicine are also bright. As we come to understand our functioning better we may learn to recognize those patterns of brain waves, muscle tension or blood pressure which eventually lead to illness. Part of a regular yearly checkup might include an analysis of these physical signs of malfunctioning before any trouble actually develops. These individuals might then be trained to deal more effectively with stress and save their bodies from needless wear and tear. We do play an active, if unknowing, part in creating many of our diseases. With the proper information and techniques we can also play an active part in preventing or correcting them.

Dr. Barbara Brown even envisions computerized self-treatment centers in every neighborhood. After an individual has been diagnosed as having an incipient illness an individualized treatment program can be prepared to correct that specific problem. He can visit his computer-doctor as often as he needs, plugging in his treatment program cassette each time, until he has learned to correct the difficulty. She has even hoped that budding neuroses and psychoses might be revealed in a brain wave analysis and corrected by brain wave training. Although admittedly quite suppositional it is likely that this possibility will be carefully explored in the next few years. With half the hospital beds in the whole country occupied by mental patients there are certain to be many scientists interested in any chance for relief for these individuals.

5

Alphacare

Mullen is a small residential avenue which runs over some of the most peaceful and sunny hills in San Francisco. The one-family wooden houses look comfortable and well kept. There are flowers in most of the yards. It is a neighborhood which likes itself and you instantly sense that it would be a good place to live. It is not the type of setting one associates with words like *breakthrough* or *wave of the future.* And yet it is somehow appropriate that one of the seeds of the future has taken root here and begun to grow.

No. 67 Mullen is the site of Nöogenesis, Inc., possibly the first legitimate biofeedback training center open to the public in the world. There is a great deal of feedback training currently being done in this country right at this moment, but it is in laboratories, universities and special schools. They are run by scientists and their primary object is research. While they once needed to pay the subjects for these experiments, individuals who are eager for the experience have volunteered in such numbers that some workers now report having lists of more than five hundred names of subjects who have offered to participate without payment. The subjects accept the fact that they will have nothing to say about the type of training they will receive, if indeed they are ever called, or even whether they will actually receive feedback training rather than be placed in a control group.

At Nöogenesis an individual may be referred by his physician or therapist for training in specific skills he needs, or he may make an appointment for himself and request help in learning to deal with a particular problem. It is headed by Frank Burns, a young psychologist with experience in both behavioral modification and electronics. Soft-spoken and well-informed, he explained that this setting was only a model for future development. Right now it is small and comfortable. Only one person can be trained at a time. There are still a number of problems to be solved before full-scale expansion would be practical.

The equipment, already extremely sophisticated, is still being refined. Frank has spent several years with some of the most creative engineers in the Bay Area helping to develop it. A full year was spent putting together the first instruments and overcoming difficult engineering problems. By the time they were completed he realized that even more must be demanded of the instruments and the work began all over again, building on what had been learned the first time. Recently his second generation of feedback equipment was finished and Nöogenesis was open to the public.

Other factors also enter into successful operation. The quiet neighborhood helps keep the training rooms free from distracting noises. Electrical interference is also moderate, but for added protection there is a hidden layer of copper mesh surrounding the entire training room. "One of the problems in using home-use machines," explained Frank, "is that they are not adequately shielded. You can pick up interference from radio and TV broadcasts, trolley cars and even household appliances. The calming and pleasant atmosphere of the neighborhood doesn't hurt either," he confided.

Frank can now get feedback and do training related to alpha waves, muscle tension, heart rate, body temperature and galvanic skin responses. The last is a measure of palm sweat which indicates degree of anxiety. The basic equipment is fully miniaturized so that it fits into a large attache case. If it were necessary he could probably make house calls. The components are also modularized so that in case of breakdown the defective circuit board could be snapped out and replacement snapped in for instant repair. Currently under development are more brain wave components to monitor delta, theta, and beta waves.

In addition to using tones for auditory feedback, the *vidium* was developed at Nöogenesis for visual feedback when indicated. The subject reclines in a large padded armchair and looks at a specially modified color television set directly in front of him. On it bright colored bands glow in the dimly lit room, each color corresponding to a different function being monitored. As he responds in the proper direction the band expands. When he is not responding the colored bar instantly shrinks. Following several functions at the same time allows for both complex learning tasks and also serves as a double and triple check on certain processes. High alpha production seems to lead almost inevitably to relaxation and reduction of anxiety. If there is any doubt, however, one can check not only the amount of alpha being produced, but also see if the heart rate is slowing, if muscles are less tense and if palm sweating has decreased.

Since they are not yet associated directly with a physician, *treatment* as such is not offered. (California law is very restrictive about the use of the word.) Rather, psycho-physiological education is offered. The distinction is more legal than actual, and in the hands of a competent individual such education can apparently help alleviate a number of problems. Frank has received offers to give seminars at medical schools in the area and expects to have a physician on the staff before too long.

Interesting results and some successes have already been accumulating despite the short time that Nöogenesis has been in full operation. Relaxation training and behavioral modification has helped one man, a homosexual, to a happier and more fulfilling life. Some male homosexuals are extremely promiscuous, often having sexual encounters with several different individuals in the same day. With relationships limited to a half hour of sex, with no intention of ever seeing the partner again, it is little wonder that they are often lonely and depressed, but the cycle is compulsive and self-sustaining. The loneliness and lack of satisfaction in casual encounters soon drives them back to the streets and bars for more contact, and more frustration.

A careful discussion with his client revealed that part of the problem was a fear of being alone. (This man had accepted his homosexuality as a part of himself and had no desire to give it up.) A short time alone in his apartment would make him anxious enough to run out to find someone, anyone, to be with. It reached a point where as soon as he left work he felt compelled to hurry to a homosexual bar for a pickup. He was miserable and wanted more from life.

Working together he and Frank developed a hierarchy to be used in relaxation training. If being alone in his apartment made him most anxious then that would be at the top of the hierarchy. At the bottom would be some point at a great psychological distance from the peak discomfort where the anxiety first began to appear in small quantities. It progresses by small psychological steps until it reached the top, or point of maximal distress.

The next step was to teach him to relax in a neutral setting with as little stimulation as possible. In the soft chair in the dimly lit room, Frank led him through a standard set of relaxation exercises while they monitored his progress on the feedback equipment. The exercises further speeded up the progress he might have made with just the feedback alone. "It's a musculo-physiological type of learning," Frank explained. "Once you get it you never forget how to do it."

After the client learned how to relax in an optimal and stress free situation they turned to the hierarchy. He would place himself in a state of deep relaxation and alpha, as verified on the vidium. Then Frank would read the lowest item on the hierarchy and the client would visualize the situation. This would introduce a note of tension and anxiety. The client would again try to relax, using his newfound skills, while he visualized the mildly stressful situation. When he could think of that setting and remain completely relaxed, they would move on to the next one, proceeding at whatever pace was most individually helpful.

Several principles were at work. One is the fact that anxiety and relaxation are mutually exclusive. You cannot be relaxed while you are anxious and vice versa. The other is the fact that although it might be difficult or impossible to deal with certain big problems all at once, small problems can usually be mastered quickly and with relative ease. The trick is to divide the big one into a whole series of small ones and take them one at a time. The steps are small and the client is faced with the same type of difficulty each time: how to master a small amount of anxiety. The distinction between thinking and doing did not appear to be a major one in this case. As he mastered various situations in his imagination during the training sessions he was also able to deal with them in his life away from the feedback situation.

The effects generalized even more than that, however. After ten weeks not only had he completed the hierarchy and was able to resist the temptations of casual and shallow relationships, but he was also able to begin a stable and intimate relationship with one person. Whenever he had tried this before he had become impotent and quickly given up. This time it did not happen and at a follow-up point some months later he was still happier, nonpromiscuous, potent and with the same person.

Also encouraging were the results of feedback training with a young woman who was in the last month of her pregnancy. The wife of a psychiatric resident realized, just a few weeks before she was due to give birth, that she was terrified of the event. With such a short time to work they embarked on a crash program, set up a hierarchy and began the sessions. They were not to have long to practice; the young woman's obstetrician apparently felt that she was somehow delaying the onset of her labor because of her anxiety (another testament to our ability to control involuntary processes) and decided to begin injections to bring on the birth. They only had time for a few training sessions and did not complete the hierarchy, but she reported that things went well and she was quite satisfied.

Limited success has also been achieved at Nöogenesis with the problem of frigidity. The sample was small, including only three women, but good results were achieved in all cases at least at first. All the women did have orgasms after training. Later two of the couples returned to their usual behavior, apparently because it was still satisfying to them for some reason, in spite of the mutual frustration it caused.

Frank became interested in new ways of helping individuals with emotional and behavioral problems because of several experiences he had. The first was eight years ago when he needed help with difficulties of his own. He tried traditional therapy and found he didn't make satisfactory progress. His therapist said it was because he wasn't trying, but he felt this wasn't true. He did want help, but he didn't know how to try. If only there were some way to show him what he had to do he would certainly do it. There wasn't any way, then. Later in his career he was teaching relaxation and deconditioning (the procedure described earlier) in California state hospitals. The relaxation was taught through the same type of exercises he now uses, but without biofeedback. He was struck by the difficulty some individuals had in spite of their motivation. The ones who needed it most seemed too tense to relax readily or well with the standard procedures. When he learned about feedback training he instantly felt that this was a meaningful breakthrough. He hasn't changed his mind since.

The Followers of Alpha

When the time arrives that alpha wave training centers finally appear in the telephone book's *Yellow Pages*, it may very likely become one of those listings with numerous cross-references. The explanation is simple—alpha is and probably will always be many things to many people; while some might look under "Religions," others may instinctively flip to "Biofeedback."

The under-thirtyish hue of most alpha adherents has already earned for alpha the image and stereotypes of "some kind of hippy thing." But, like most images and sterotypes, it is simply not true. In this chapter we shall see that the wide range of people tuning in on their alpha waves has already encompassed a far greater scope than simply drug freaks or meditationists.

Alpha, Now!

It is now history that the free-speech movement began in the San Francisco area, and that the hippie love generation was born and died here. San Francisco is the city where new and way out things get their start. Into this kind of environment came the free universities, spawning grounds for the turned off generation. So it isn't particularly surprising that a course of alpha brain waves would be offered first at a free university.

Because of the nature of free universities around the country, courses taught are generally highly unorthodox. They are rarely the kind of subjects found at the established universities. Macrame, Zen, organic cooking and, now, alpha are as natural a part of the curriculum as are physics, psychology and chemistry at the conventional institutions.

The first course in alpha waves was scheduled for instruction in 1969. But it ran into some complications before it ever got off the ground. The instructor had hoped to teach a course relating studies of alpha to ESP. He contacted Emerson Stafford, founder and director of the now defunct Entropy University. Preparations were made to offer alpha for instruction. The prompt enthusiasm for the course was reflected by the fact that enrollment quickly swelled to twenty-five (a high number for a new course, especially in late 1969, before alpha became a hip word).

But then problems came. Just days before the beginning of the two month series, the class was abruptly cancelled. The instructor, it seemed, was also employed by a scientific organization involved in a project measuring brain wave response to ordinary stimuli. His employer feared that he would be revealing methodological techniques which he did not want made public. Consequently, the instructor was given an ultimatum: Drop the course or be fired.

That specific course, then, was never taught. This development was particularly unfortunate, not only because Entropy lost a potentially valuable class, but also because the correlation between alpha and ESP is a scientific matter which is now undergoing serious exploration. The data turned out by the course would certainly have been interesting.

A new course, with a new instructor, finally made the Entropy catalog in early 1970. The particular focus of this course, rather than ESP, was biofeedback—an analysis of what sort of signals come from the brain. The alpha state was included in the studies. The course drew fifteen students.

Jules Geib, one of the fifteen, felt that he and most of his classmates went into the course with little specific knowledge of what would happen. He reported that the group discussions drifted rather freely, generally focusing on the nervous system, brain waves and sensory input. Each week several students, on a rotating basis, would monitor their own alpha waves through alpha feedback machines. By the end of the eight weekly sessions each participant had several opportunities to check out his or her alpha. And here the class made a very interesting observation which has cropped up in studies of alpha. It was observed that about half of the students enrolled seemed to show generally better results with alpha than the others. And it was these same people who were also involved with Zen meditation. Their findings seemed to coincide with the results of the alpha studies of Japanese Buddhists cited earlier. The alpha output of class members who practiced meditation showed more frequent and longer enduring alpha output than others in the group.

The highlight of the course occurred at the last session with a visit to the laboratory of Dr. Joseph Kamiya (alpha's Freud). Here the students had the opportunity of repeating their alpha checks in the same laboratory where much of the alpha research was pioneered. Each participant was studied for alpha. And, again in Dr. Kamiya's laboratory, it was noted that the results tended to parallel the Japanese studies. That is, Zen and meditation practitioners show a propensity for turning on alpha with greater frequency and more sustained periods of time.

Zen and Alpha

In further exploring the link between alpha and Zen we were fortunate in being able to visit a center for Zen studies. Silas Hoadley is thirty-two years old and an assistant Zen teacher and senior student who has been studying at the San Francisco Zen Center for eight years. During the past four years he has participated in three experiments which were related to brain waves. We will discuss these experiments shortly.

At the Zen Center, the experience began as we entered the building. We were greeted at the door and cordially invited into the inner patio courtyard where most of the sixty-five male and female residents had gathered for afternoon tea and cake. Shortly after the refreshments were served everyone rose, made a Buddhist bow and began reciting Buddhist verses in unison. Recitation and personal meditation, as we later discovered, are integral parts of their daily lives.

The physical milieu within the Zen Center is one of calmness and serenity. Flowers and plants are in abundance. The rooms are spacious, with high ceilings and muted colors. The floors are covered with mats, which are for the meditation exercises; a peaceful quiet pervades the entire building.

Several years prior to joining the Zen Center, Silas Hoadley had experimented with psychedelic drugs. He found, however, that drugs did not provide full answers. He was quick to assure us that drugs are no part of the practices carried out at the Center.

Within the past few years, Zen Center students have participated in three alpha brain wave experiments conducted under the auspices of Dr. Kamiya and Langley Porter Neuropsychiatric Institute. On one occasion Dr. Kamiya's assistants wheeled EEG machines into the center, hoping to chart the brain waves of Hoadley in his familiar environment.

When in *zazen*, the traditional sitting position for meditation, Hoadley was measured for alpha. The monitoring took place over a period of several hours. The procedure was repeated at a later date, but this time Hoadley was checked for alpha output while sleeping. At this point Hoadley has not yet been informed as to the results of the sessions, but he is aware that Dr. Kamiya has also researched other meditation groups. No one really knows what such studies of alpha and meditation can or will lead to. It is possible that alpha researchers may find additional data linking meditation to alpha waves. If the link also extends to the phenomenon of sleep as well, then the enigma becomes all the more interesting. Hoadley says, "It may not be anything new as a phenomenon of the meditation mind but, scientifically, it just is not yet clearly understood."

Dr. Kamiya's research carried out with the Zen Center was the only contact most of the students at the Center ever had with either an EEG or alpha machine. One exception was a 65-year-old Zen student whose enthusiasm for the new seemed to be without limits—he had made an attempt at introducing alpha machines into the Center's training, but his idea was met with apathy.

Nevertheless, it appears that the futures of alpha and Zen may very well be bound up with each other. It has already been speculated, mostly in the popular magazines, that alpha is a short cut to the state of Zen meditation for which the Masters often spend many years. Some project the possibility of telescoping thousands of years of Zen into a few hours on the alpha machine—a form of instant Zen. (Hoadley recalls a similar widespread enthusiasm for LSD when it became readily available on the streets. Suddenly LSD was hailed as a way to instant wisdom.) Undoubtedly some people who are in search of self-fulfillment, upon reading this book, will want to purchase one of the numerous alpha machines available on the market.

Hoadley would not purchase an alpha machine, and he would have his doubts about anybody claiming to be seriously studying Zen primarily with the help of a machine. He feels that such students would most likely be ambivalent about their own involvement in Zen and, he adds, "They inevitably run into a certain point of their own resistance. Zen training implies total unconditioning. Alpha training goes only part way; there has to be more than just mental or cerebral involvement."

Hoadley sees a possibility that alpha will bring some potential students to Zen practice. If alpha does develop as part of modern cultural technology Zen students will undoubtedly try it and develop some capacity to control and manipulate various body-mind functions.

Hoadley feels, however, that if students become seriously involved with alpha training they will soon find its limitations. And he succinctly points out, "Students will then discover that they're flogging a dead horse. They've learned to relax somewhat but they're still left with their basic life situation."

Contrary to what the reader may surmise from the above, alpha machines are not necessarily in conflict with Zen according to Hoadley. However he expresses concern for the Zen student who may begin to rely too heavily on the alpha machine. "I feel that using an alpha machine would hinder the mind less than massive doses of, say, drugs or coffee before entering a meditation period. I think that the only real hindrance would be if a dependency on technique were formed."

Hoadley has no objections to students using alpha machines, as long as it is kept apart from the study of Zen. "If a student wants to use it, fine. But he shouldn't force it on the practice itself." For himself, he is interested in understanding alpha training as he knows that the phenomenon is upcoming. But he feels no urgency or desire to use a feedback machine himself, as he thinks that Zen practice is fundamentally thorough.

A Zen student must be aware of much going on from within his body. To integrate this awareness he must go through a process of exposing the self to the body's biological functions. For example, zazen is a period of vivid relaxation and readiness with no particular object held in mind. The spine is kept straight and the breathing is generally deep. This is the state in which Zen masters have been observed to yield high outputs of alpha. It may be that in this state the alpha rhythm is the product of calm, relaxed awakeness emanating from alert composure. When these traits are developed there is a greater likelihood of higher yields of alpha.

Alpha and Religion: Compatible?

Getting into an alpha state is nothing phenomenal for the Zen enthusiast. As we have just seen, alpha seems to be an integral part of the whole Zen experience. A question arises, however, over what enticement alpha holds for those who are raised with traditional Western beliefs. After our meeting at the Zen Center we were curious to meet someone from the Judeo-Christian tradition who could perhaps answer this question. The opportunity came sometime later when we met Sister Mary Alma, director of the Library Science Program at the University of San Francisco.

After talking to her for only a short time, we discovered she is really one of the most interesting and varied personalities we had come across in our alpha studies.

For many years Sister Alma has been an avid reader of science fiction. She has attended numerous science fiction symposiums and conventions and has met some of the foremost writers of science fiction in this country. She has always been interested in the natural power of extrasensory perception. For her the world of the supernatural does not have the fear and apprehension most people feel. She accepts the existence of extraterrestial beings and strongly believes that UFO's are not merely figments of people's imagination.

In recent months Sister Alma has become a true believer in alpha. For her alpha holds the promise of answering certain problems which affect both individuals and society as a whole. She sees no contradiction between alpha and her faith. Sister Alma believes that making use of alpha is merely one way of tapping the potential of the body God has given to man. Since alpha is within the realm of man, it is therefore within his power to seek this experience.

Sister Alma attributes her initial interest in exploring powers of the mind to books she read on hypnotism and mind control while recuperating from an operation. Gradually her interest drifted toward alpha. For this reason, when invited to do so, Sister attended a Mind Dynamics weekend workshop being taught on controlling one's own mind. Despite some criticisms that have been directed toward the mind schools,

Sister feels that the Mind Dynamics course is basically sound. She sees that these types of group experiences are bringing people together as they begin to communicate with each other. For many persons, she believes, the alpha experience may lead to a renaissance of personal development and to an increase in self-satisfaction. "We all have the capability," Sister says, "of improving the functioning of our mind. The problem is that we have not yet developed this potential."

For Sister Alma, developing mind power is one of the keys to living a fuller and more satisfying existence. And, looking to the future, she sees alpha as the method by which the human potential for ESP might be developed.

Although Sister Alma has never been monitored by the electroencephalograph machine, she feels confident that she is able to enter the alpha state at will, simply by going through the proper thought process; she reports that she has been able to incorporate this ability to the betterment of her daily life. When fatigued, for example, she will enter a state of alpha for barely a few minutes and emerge feeling as if she had napped for an hour. She also is able to cool herself down upon walking into an overheated room, simply by going into an alpha level. Since birth, Sister has had difficulties with her back which, from time to time, have caused a great deal of suffering. But by getting into an alpha state she is able to suppress the pain.

Sister Alma believes in alpha control. At this time it is not really known to what extent other members of the clergy have responded with this kind of interest. It is not inconceivable, however, that youth groups, such as the Jesus freaks, might begin to use alpha as part of their *being*. Whether the more established religious groups in our society do the same remains to be seen.

Group Alpha

The popularization of alpha has finally brought it to the marketplace; like many other things in the United States, alpha services can now be purchased. Alpha House, directed by Shirley Crane, a former Communications instructor at San Francisco State College, is one of these budding organizations.

Sessions at Alpha House are offered in a series of four group meetings which are stretched over a period of two weeks. The total cost for ten hours is $20. Miss Crane sees Alpha House as a place where each participant will learn to recognize his own alpha state, first through the use of a machine, and eventually progress to a level where feedback (and therefore the machine) is no longer needed. "A prime advantage of attending Alpha House," says Miss Crane, "is that instead of buying expensive alpha equipment that the user may soon outgrow, the alpha student need only spend a minimum of time and money to achieve his or her goal of alpha control." Miss Crane adds that the ultimate goal of Alpha House is to enable each practitioner to produce the alpha rhythm at any time, any place, at will.

Alpha House was a long time in the making, the result of a great deal of research and preparation. For Miss Crane the purpose of training individuals to attain the alpha state comes down to a single goal—relaxation. "Profound relaxation," she states, "generated not by drugs but by biofeedback trained self-awareness and self-control is a big step in learning to relate better to ourselves and to the world."

Increasing numbers of people are using the alpha machine in the privacy of their own surroundings. But now the concept of group participation adds interesting possibilities and dynamics to the alpha experience. Attending one of these group sessions at Alpha House, we found much to be said for the seriousness and intent which seems to characterize the two and a half hour sessions.

The atmosphere is jovial. But once the actual alpha monitoring begins, conversation stops, and the lights are dimmed. The group members spend the session reclining on large pillows which are scattered about the room. From this position each member spends an hour attempting to put his mind in the state of alpha. During this time Miss Crane, unnoticed by the students, monitors the alpha output of each individual by means of an earphone which is plugged into wires that lead from each of the alpha sets. (Lest anyone be confused, the group members are not attempting to communicate with Miss Crane or each other. Rather, each individual is producing his own alpha for himself.)

At the conclusion of the first hour, Miss Crane gives each member feedback on his or her own alpha output. Then the group members discuss their feelings and problems related to alpha—what did and did not succeed in enhancing their entering the alpha state; did changing the position of the electrodes (from the occipital to the frontal lobes) have any effect on alpha output? Achievement of alpha is really something of a trial and error process in which the variables may be as personal as one's own private thoughts. Miss Crane finds this method of group discussion to be an effective means by which the participants "build up vibrations within the group of alpha production."

Not everyone is initially able to produce high outputs of alpha; for some it may require the entire ten hours' training to show any results. Others seem able to achieve the alpha state almost immediately. One student at Alpha House reported an inability to sleep one night following an alpha session. He became so relaxed and stimulated from the session that sleep was not necessary.

The first couple of times Kathleen Fornason hooked herself up at Alpha House she was a failure—the headset tone was irritating, she was bored and she had no alpha output. But when Kathleen finally succeeded sometime later in producing alpha it was no great surprise to her. Her sensitivity training experiences at San Francisco State College had made her aware of her own body and had given her the ability to relax, thus enhancing alpha.

Kathleen really isn't atypical of people attracted to alpha. She more or less drifted into acting, receiving a bachelor's degree in drama, and is now working on a master's degree in Broadcast Communication Arts. She says that her enthusiasm for alpha comes from a keen interest in the mind and a desire to know about current trends. "In broadcasting you have to know about what's going on, the fads, what's happening to people."

These two women are conducting some experiments in correlating alpha output and piano playing (Kathleen has studied the piano since childhood). The idea came to them after Kathleen mentioned that when she is playing the piano her mind is focusing on one thing only—the music. Their hypothesis is that when Kathleen, or any pianist, is past the point of struggle, ceases to be concerned with individual notes and is able to flow and be at one with the music, then the pianist will be in the state of alpha.

While most of the patrons at Alpha House find that the group experience works to their benefit, there are those who find it something of an impediment. Individuals who are particularly shy, or ill at ease in groups, often find it difficult to achieve the state of relaxation which is essential to good alpha. Occasionally initial failure tempts one to the state where he is "trying" to produce alpha; this invariably will lead to low levels of output or none at all.

The experience of Alpha House seems to indicate that alpha is a highly individual experience, whether the participant is in a group or on his own. Presently Alpha House is unique. Its success and the enthusiasm it has generated seems to hold the promise of even greater expansion. Hopefully it will do so without the cost of its charm.

The Awareness Lab

Another of the newly budding alpha-oriented business enterprises is one operated by Norman Sturgis, dramatist and writer. Sturgis runs Theatre-Media Lab in Mill Valley, California, which he instructs twice weekly. From here he has drawn a good deal of his philosophy as it relates to alpha. A basic theme of his instruction is the concept of relaxing and being at ease with one's self in order to produce freely and creatively. For this reason many of his students are encouraged to explore the alpha experience.

In the twenty-five years in which Sturgis has been involved with the theater he has studied numerous concepts of communication. He feels that this has given him a keen awareness of how creativity, mental calmness and self-assurance contribute to the process of acting. *States of being* have been a part of his profession for twenty-five years; his exploration of alpha merely carries it further by another step.

Recently Mr. Sturgis purchased a PSI 360 alpha set. Hoping to return some of his investment, and spread the experience of alpha, he placed an ad in a large newspaper announcing that anyone interested in monitoring their brain waves and increasing alpha production should contact him at the Awareness Lab. At this time, he reports that there has been a rather brisk response. He offers individual appointments to interested callers, who pay a fee which may range from $3 to $5 per session, depending on the number of sessions.

The training sessions are held in his own home, amidst a relaxed business-like atmosphere. Tacked onto a bulletin board is a typewritten page which gives a brief description of alpha and what the student should expect from his early experiences.

Most of Sturgis' contacts are interested primarily in trying out the machine on a one-time-only basis. Some, however, have taken such an interest that they have ended up purchasing a machine of their own.

Situated high on a hill covered with trees, the location in Mill Valley of Sturgis' Awareness Lab seems as if it were chosen with the idea of encouraging high output of alpha. The facility itself is a cozy, five-room cottage. A den, adjacent to the living room, has been set off solely for the use of his alpha customers. His equipment represents an investment of a substantial amount of money.

Mounted above an easy chair is an electronic device which connects the alpha headset to an amplifier. This, in turn, amplifies the oscillations on a loudspeaker so others in the room may hear the alpha output as the individual monitors himself with the headset. Another set of wires goes from the headset to an oscilloscope. When the user is hooked up to the oscilloscope and is producing alpha, his wave patterns appear on the scope as rising and falling blips.

Some of the equipment occasionally creates problems for the beginner. For example, to use the oscilloscope the eyes must be open. And in the case of beginners there is always the problem of visual distraction preventing the user from achieving a constant alpha wave. Thus most beginners prefer to continue their alpha output with auditory feedback only. Once they master this mode they can progress to opening the eyes.

Often in the process of his home sessions, Sturgis will record the brain wave patterns on a tape recorder. He sends the tapes to a laboratory where they are analyzed by a computer for the various brain wave levels. His present focus of interest, aside from alpha, is in a wave called theta (believed to have some correlation to the creative process).

Since Sturgis has been offering his services, the makeup of his clients has ranged from school teachers to businessmen to a writer of TV commercials. Some, no doubt, are drawn by simple curiosity, while others see alpha as an answer to their own particular needs. One businessman had been hoping to use the alpha experience to increase his business, but the results did not please him. Another found himself extremely nervous, but after an alpha trial he complained, "When I'm putting out alpha, I can't think." This disturbed him and he quit. (Incidentally, Sturgis reports that for some unknown reason businessmen seem to be members of a "low alpha" profession.)

Another of Sturgis' clients, a woman, claimed that she had great difficulties being around people due to anxieties she felt in social situations. The Sturgis technique combined alpha control with old-fashioned Skinner box psychology. A light box was set up with a picture of people taped to a translucent panel. The word *people* was written across the picture. Once the client puts on the headset and begins slipping into the pleasant, relaxed state of alpha, the people-picture flashes, thereby creating an association between the concept of people and a simultaneously pleasant alpha experience. The client claims that it works and she plans to keep coming until her problem is resolved completely.

Most of Sturgis' clients are professionals. They are young, usually ranging in age between twenty-five and thirty-five. Their statements about post-alpha observations range from mild euphoria to increased pleasures at making love. One individual, a school teacher, claims that she finds herself very relaxed, sometimes to the point of a carefree attitude on her job.

Although the research director for Medlab of San Francisco, an upcoming producer of alpha machines, didn't participate in Awareness Lab, his responses to the alpha effect complement those of the schoolteacher just cited. He has found alpha control to be very useful for regaining composure during tense business meetings or in the middle of trying to solve a difficult problem. This gentleman states: "It's like counting to ten when you're mad—in this case you've added the assurance that you are consciously switching into alpha." Occasionally he goes one step further in combining alpha with self-hypnosis. He has found the combination to be of help in getting into the proper state of mind to do tasks at hand.

Alpha is many things to many people—some want to be successful, others want to enhance their ability to communicate. But for Bob Nelson, a rehabilitation counselor, experiences with alpha have led him to believe in its potential value for psychiatric therapy. Nelson described his own thoughts as being in the realm of therapeutic goals. He believes that some clients will be able to achieve the same pervading sense of calmness that he himself has experienced. "I'm in alpha when things are flowing. It's there when I'm not being subjected to unnecessary friction, such as hassles with other people. Alpha," he says, "is being so much in control that I can let go of the idea of control. I float freely; it's an experience of being into 'Now.' Alpha means to become one with yourself."

NOTE TO THE READER

Some research in the field of alpha brain waves and biofeedback indicates the possibility of physical and/or medical harm and danger to the user of alpha and biofeedback machines. This can occur from improper assembly and malfunctioning of a machine. It is strongly urged that you have your complete kit checked out by a qualified electronics expert before using it. The authors, publishers, or their agents assume no responsibility for assembly, functioning, usage, or problems arising from equipment.

7

Building Your Own Biofeedback Machines

The purchase of commercial biofeedback instruments is presently plagued with pitfalls. Since the biofeedback boom in the popular press, numerous instrument companies have sprung up. The quality of the devices produced by some of these companies for amplifying, filtering and feeding back bio-signals has been rather poor. It would appear that in some instances these manufacturers have spent more time, money and effort in preparing speculative sales advertisements than in the design and construction of their instruments. While some hints will be provided to help you in selecting a suitable biofeedback device, if you wish to purchase one, you will stand a far better chance of limiting your risk and expense if you decide to build your own from the diagrams provided in this chapter.

A great deal of concern has been expressed by the Society for Psychophysiological Research over the unrestricted manufacture and sale of biofeedback instruments to the public. The Society fears these are of inferior quality (*e.g.*, EEG instruments which respond to muscle artifacts with a feedback signal) and sold with extravagant claims ranging from increasing sexual potency to eliminating phobias. Similar concern over the unrestricted sale of the more than two dozen alpha brain wave biofeedback devices now on the market has led the U.S. Food and Drug Administration to consider taking regulatory action. If successful in their efforts the FDA would require all feedback devices to pass inspection standards appropriate for regulating medical devices. Further federal regulation may ultimately bring biofeedback equipment under the umbrella of prescription items, available only through special grants or a physician's signature.

Such regulation is certain to be controversial. On the one hand there is a greater likelihood of higher instrument quality. Similarly, the rules for truth-in-advertising about the uses and effects of various forms of feedback will probably be more carefully observed. On the other hand a lessening of accessibility to the feedback experience may ensue. Significantly fewer members of the lay public will be able to purchase biofeedback equipment or become involved in personal experimentation with body self-control. As such restrictions reach their zenith even scientists may find it difficult to freely study biofeedback phenomena, much as research on LSD and marijuana has been significantly limited. The net effect may be a reduction in fruitful investigation and application in the biofeedback area.

It is doubtful whether many scientists, at this point, have cause for alarm as they often employ laboratory technicians who are skilled in electronics and equipment construction. Thus, they usually custom-build biofeedback equipment suited to their own special needs. However, since few of us are scientists it is the general public which may be most affected by federal regulation of biofeedback equipment.

At present there are still three broad alternatives for personal experimentation with biofeedback: (1) buy biofeedback equipment already on the market, (2) participate in biofeedback experiments at universities as a subject, and (3) build your own equipment.

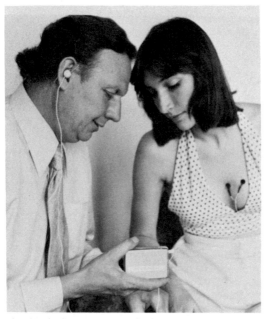

Although galvanic skin response biofeedback monitors do not directly measure alpha brain waves, the above machine is an example of how compact and portable some biofeedback devices can be constructed. This battery-operated model, small enough to fit in the palm, monitors skin responses through several finger tip or body (shown above) electrodes. (Photo courtesy of Eidetic Consultants Limited, Toronto, Canada.)

At this time no less than thirty separate biofeedback instrument manufacturers have come into existence. Devices for alpha training have been most popular with interest in other brain waves rapidly gaining. For the home investigator, however, other forms of feedback experimentation, notably galvanic skin responses, can be relatively simple, inexpensive and quite rewarding.

The price for EEG feedback devices range from about $35 to $600, the average price being about $200. Prices for these machines have dropped into the consumer range largely because of the development of the integrated circuit. An integrated circuit (IC) is a complex circuit which is pre-wired and packaged as a single unit (usually smaller than a dime) which can be joined with other ICs and used in producing stereo amplifiers, EEGs, computers, etc. The popularity and usefulness of these tiny circuits has led to their being mass-produced, which has driven their cost down markedly. A current example of their effect on prices is seen in electronic pocket calculators and digital wristwatches.

In general the same rules apply to biofeedback equipment that would apply to the purchase of any major electronic appliance. Are there any warranties or guarantees? How long does the company stand behind their product? Is there a branch office in your area? Are there service representatives through another company? Are the equipment specifications spelled out? Do they provide adequate instructions? Just because you are buying a scientific instrument doesn't mean that you won't be subjected to the same type of sales techniques which are used to sell automobiles, washing machines and car stereos. It is easy to fall into the trap of buying from the company which seems to make the greatest claims regarding feedback effects. But effects vary from person to person and depend much more on the application of the device, given the fact that you have an instrument which reports biological changes back to you accurately and reliably.

Luckily there is a simple formula that may be used in purchasing the best alpha wave machine. It requires answering four simple questions, in addition to those posed beforehand about a manufacturer's reliability and service.

The basic questions are:

1. *What type of electrodes are provided?*
   a. Stainless steel are worst
   b. Disposable silver—silver chloride better
   c. Permanent silver—silver chloride are best

Distortion is minimized with the improved electrodes. Electrode noise and electrode long-term drift is optimum with "c" electrodes.

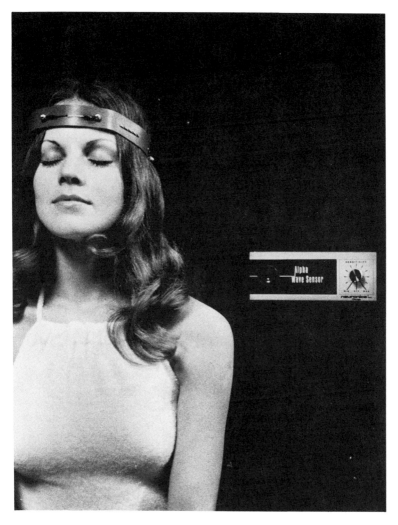

A majority of the brain wave monitoring devices on the market measure
both alpha and theta brain waves. Electrodes implanted in the headband
in this model pick up the brain waves and the electronic circuit transforms
them into audible tones. (Photo courtesy of Neuronics, Inc., Chicago, Ill.)

2. *What is the common mode rejection?*
   a. Less than 40 d is intolerable in most cities
   b. 60 d is better
   c. 80 d and up is best.

The common mode rejection (CMR) relates to how well the device rejects strong electric fields and radiation from 60 Hz power lines. Low CMR places serious demands on filters, and further distorts signals from the brain. Poor CMR leads to "hum" mixed with the feedback signal.

3. *How many controls are provided?*
   a. Two (sensitivity and volume) is a bare minimum
   b. Three (sensivitity, volume and integration—direct or averaged) is better
   c. Five and up (sensitivity, volume, integration— direct or averaged, modulation, threshold, band select) is best.

The controls provided give an indication of the flexibility of the device. Feedback controls are the most important. Next, is there some form of calibration on the sensitivity control for recording daily improvement?

4. *What is the differential input resistance for brain waves?*
   a. 100K ohms is minimum
   b. 1M ohm is good
   c. megohm (meg) and up is best

Input resistance attenuates the brain wave signal. It forces more gain in the amplifiers. As it gets lower, excessive gain is required which leads to poor dampening and instability.

To answer these questions you need to compare the manufacturer's data sheet for the four items. If you can't get the manufacturer's data sheet forget them—they must be either hiding a poor design behind slick claims or you're too lazy to squeeze it out of them.

Upon receiving the data sheets, you need to sit down and compare them, then look at costs. You'll be amazed.

Fortunately, a lot of this work has already been done for you. In a paper submitted to the *American Psychologist*, "Of Bread, Circuses and Alpha Machines," Robert L. Schwitzgebel

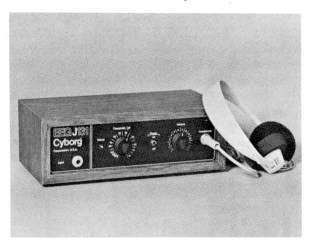

This brain wave training unit sends the monitored feedback signals into headphones which the user wears. Some units on the market, such as the above, also have a meter or light indicator to visually indicate the yielding of specific brain wave frequencies. (Photo courtesy of Cyborg Corporation, Boston, Massachusetts.)

and John D. Rugh of Claremont Graduate School provide a comparative table of 12 alpha machines costing under $200. The results speak for themselves. The journal is available at any large library.

It will be helpful to remember that the tiny electric currents produced by the brain, which we call brain waves, are considered to be difficult physiological events to monitor accurately. They are highly susceptible to both environmental and human changes; they vary from day to day and require rather complex equipment for measurement. These factors, combined with the novice's limited knowledge of how the central nervous system functions, make for certain difficulties in learning to produce and control alpha initially. Take comfort in the fact that even experienced scientists quite frequently run into recording difficulties.

You may wish to begin biofeedback exploration with one of the less complex systems. The galvanic skin response (GSR) requires relatively simple and inexpensive equipment and is

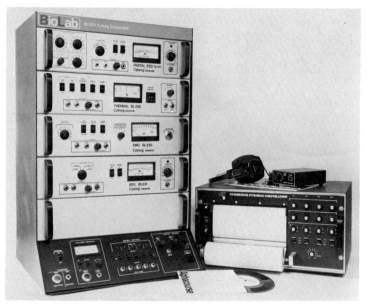

Complex feedback laboratories, as above, are designed more for the serious researcher or professional than the novice. Such units are capable of simultaneously monitoring various physiological functions to give a total profile of the subject. (Photo courtesy of Cyborg Corporation, Boston, Massachusetts.)

not difficult to work with. The GSR is a change in the skin's resistance to the passage of a weak electrical current. The change, partly due to sweating, is an aspect of the body's physiochemical response to emotional stimuli. Generally speaking, the more the body responds emotionally the less electrical resistance it offers. The current is much too mild to be detected by the subject and gives no discomfort. This measure is quite sensitive to anxiety and can be used, with appropriate feedback, in anxiety-reduction training. The reported effects on consciousness of decreasing the number of GSRs and increasing skin resistance have in some instances been similar to the alpha state of relaxation and freedom from tension.

It is hoped that the relatively uncomplex GSR circuits will allow the electronic hobbyist to make an inexpensive (approximately $25) GSR feedback device. Before beginning the task of building electronic instruments it is a good idea to have some useful references close at hand. The following are recommended.

P. H. Venables and Irene Martin, eds.
A Manual of Psychophysiological Methods
New York: American Elsevier, 1967.

Stuart A. Hoenig and Leland Payne
Electronics Without Pain: The HiFi Scientist's Guide to Applications of Electronics
Boston: Little Brown and Co., 1973

J. A. Stanley
Electronics for the Beginner, 2nd ed.
Indianapolis: Howard W. Sams & Co., 1973

Walter Schott, Coordinating Editor
Fascinating Electronic Projects for Under $10.00 Calectro Electronics
Rockford, Ill.: Hydrometals, Inc., 1973

Mitchell Waite
Projects in Sight, Sound & Sensation
Indianapolis: Howard W. Sams & Co., 1974

The device diagramed below provides a visual feedback signal from a meter whenever a sharp change in resistance occurs.

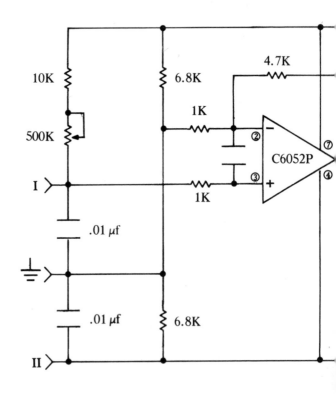

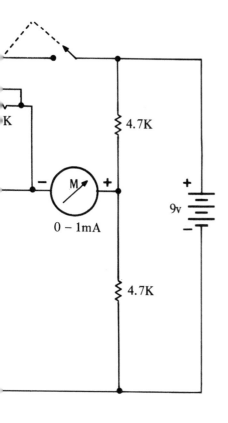

In this configuration the subject's skin resistance makes up one leg of the bridge (Wheatstone bridge) while resistors make up the other side of the bridge. When a small voltage is applied across the bridge any change in the subject's resistance will be seen as a differential voltage which is amplified by the operational amplifier (OP AMP, C 6052 P).

The general idea of the Wheatstone bridge circuit is seen below.

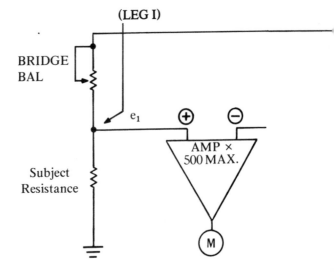

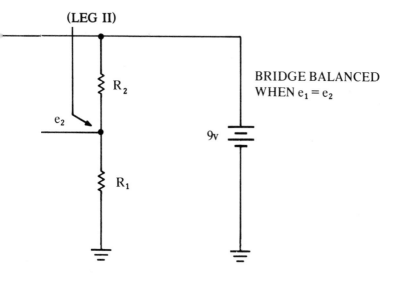

(LEG II)

R_2

e_2

R_1

9v

BRIDGE BALANCED
WHEN $e_1 = e_2$

This simple but very useful circuit has many variations. The above representation illustrates how the voltage within the system can be made stable, causing no deflection to ultimately occur with the meter (M). Then when the subject's resistance changes sharply it causes a differential voltage to occur between leg I and leg II of the bridge. This differential is amplified by the OP AMP and read as a meter deflection (feedback).

Thus, this circuit involves mechanisms which force the subject's initial resting basal skin resistance to be nulled or balanced to zero. If, for example, the subject's basal resistance is 40 kilohms, which represents one leg of the bridge, a variable resistor is adjusted to approximate the 40 kilohms balancing the meter. As sharp changes in resistance on the subject's skin occur (*e.g.*, when tense, apprehensive or startled by unexpected stimuli) the difference in the subject's initial resistance from his basal resistance unbalances the bridge, causing a meter deflection which serves as the biofeedback signal.

The parts for building this circuit are as follows:

QUANTITY	DESCRIPTION
3	Capacitors, 0.01 mfd
1	Resistor, 10 kohm
2	Resistors, 6.8 kohm
2	Resistors, 1 kohm
3	Resistors, 4.7 kohm
1	Op, amp, Motorola #HEP C6052P (IC)
1	Panel meter, 1 ma
1	Potentiometer, 500 K linear
1	Potentiometer with switch, 500 K
1	Phenolic case
2	Knobs
1	Battery connector
3	Banana jacks
3	Banana plugs
1 pkg.	Shielded audio cable, 8 ft.
1	Perforated board
1	Mine mount (for IC)
1	9-volt battery

Although the subject of electrodes can pose serious problems in scientific research, on GSR activity it need not be a major consideration for our purposes. Hydrometals, Inc., suggest that adequate electrodes can be made from a pair of bicycle trouser bands. After the bands are sanded to free them of lacquer and corrosion they can be clipped easily on the palms of the hands. It will be necessary to attach these clips to cables which connect to banana plugs for insetting into the GSR box. Shielded audio cable can serve this purpose quite well. The wire cord of the cable is soldered on one side to the electrode and on the other side to the banana plug. The outer wire shielding is intertwined from both pieces of cable and soldered to the third banana plug. Remember to dry the palms of the hands before attaching the electrodes.

It should be mentioned that although this GSR is simple to build, the ensuing results are controversial at the scientific level. Consider the fact that to balance the bridge, a current must be passed through the subject. What is the effect on the subject from this offset current? Consider that the bridge, and hence display, is highly nonlinear; resistance variations will be different as base subject resistance slowly drifts.

With these considerations in mind, a GSR such as this can show very interesting displays of gross physiological subject resistance variations.

If you're a real "do-it-yourselfer" you might want to consider a set of published plans on how to build your own alpha wave biofeedback monitor. An article appearing in the January 1973 issue of *Popular Electronics*, "Alpha Brain Wave Feedback Monitor," details the operation and construction of a high-performance EEG feedback monitor. A kit of parts and an assembly manual for the monitor can also be purchased through the article. *Popular Electronics* is carried by most libraries. For illustration purposes the schematic of the alpha machine is reproduced with the permission of the author. Only the well-experienced experimenter, however, should attempt construction without first reading the entire PE article.

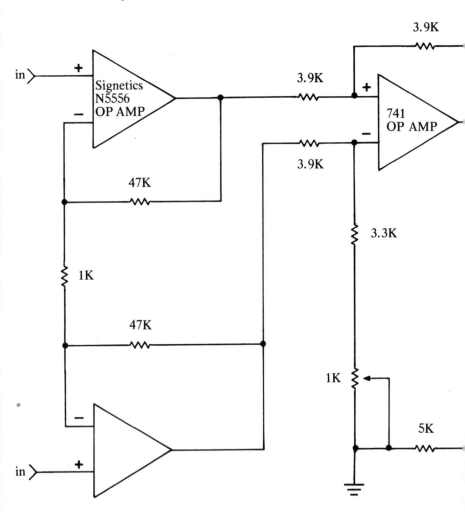

INPUT AMPLIFIERS

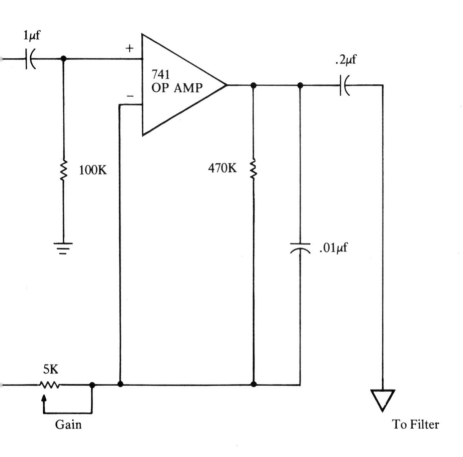

(Printed with the kind permission
of Mitchell Waite.)

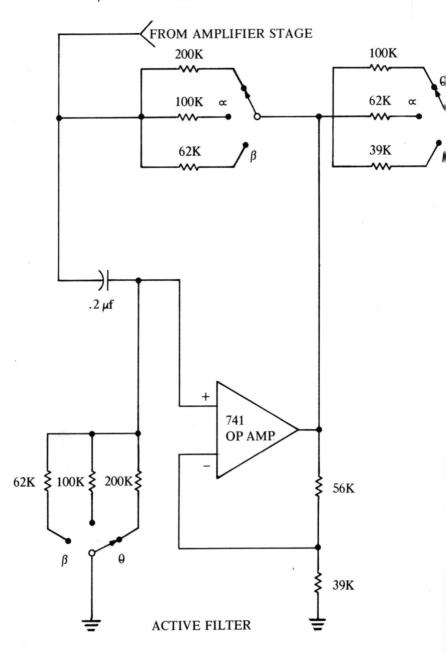

(Printed with the kind permission of Mitchell Waite.)

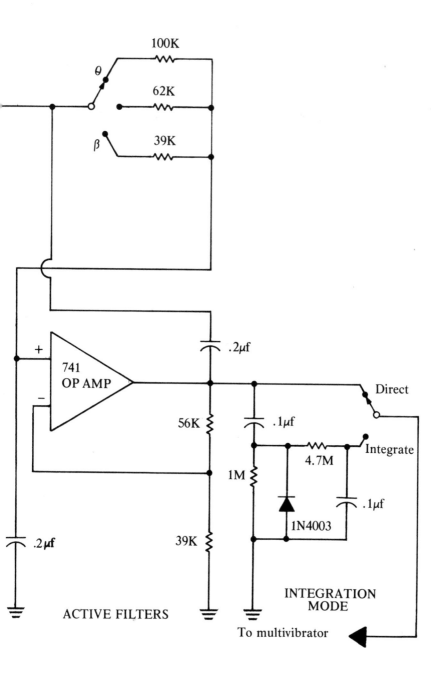

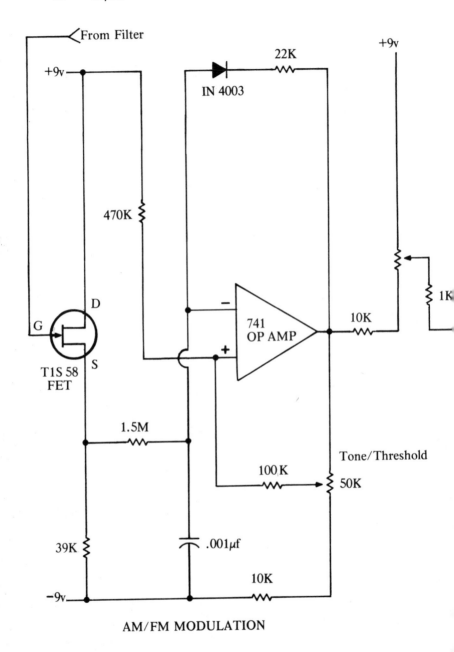

AM/FM MODULATION

(Printed with the kind permission of Mitchell Waite.)

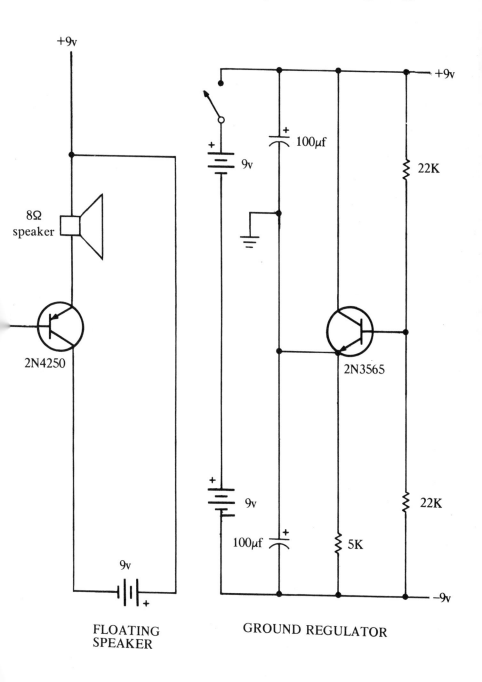

+9v

8Ω
speaker

2N4250

9v

FLOATING
SPEAKER

+9v

100μf

9v

22K

2N3565

9v

100μf

5K

22K

−9v

GROUND REGULATOR

An approximate parts list for the EEG feedback circuit is as follows:

QUANTITY	DESCRIPTION
3	9-volt battery
1	Signal capacitor, 1 mfg, 10%
1	Disc. capacitor, .01 mfg.
4	Mylar capacitor, .2 mfg., 10%
2	Mylar capacitor, .1 mfg., 10%
1	Mylar capacitor, .0001 mfg., 10%
2	Electrolytic capacitor, 100 mfg., 2 volt
2	Silicone diode, IN4003
2	OP AMP, N5556 (signetics)
5	OP AMP, 741
1	FET, TIS58
1	Transistor 2N4250
1	Transistor 2N3565
2	Resistor, 1K, ¼ watt, 5%
2	Resistor, 47K ¼ watt, 5%
3	Resistor, 3.9K, ¼ watt, 5%
1	Resistor, 3.3K, ¼ watt, 5%
6	Resistor, 100K, ¼ watt, 5%
2	Resistor, 470K, ¼ watt, 5%
2	Resistor, 5K, ¼ watt, 5%
4	Resistor, 62K, ¼ watt, 5%
2	Resistor, 200K, ¼ watt, 5%
2	Resistor, 56K, ¼ watt, 5%
5	Resistor, 39K, ¼ watt, 5%
1	Resistor, 1M, ¼ watt, 5%
1	Resistor, 4.7M, ¼ watt, 5%
1	Resistor, 1.5M, ¼ watt, 5%
3	Resistor, 10K. ¼ watt, 5%
1	Speaker, 8 ohm

Once constructed, it is possible to feed back not only alpha, but beta (above 15 Hz) and theta (5-7 Hz) brain waves with this device.

This particular set of EEG circuits has several advantages usually found in very expensive equipment. For instance, 4-pole band pass filters tuned to the center frequency of alpha, theta and beta allow for identification of these low frequency, narrow band wave forms. The type of auditory feedback is also an important consideration. These circuits include features such as the direct/integrate switch which determines which part of the brain wave will vary the tone. In the direct setting the instantaneous brain wave which passes through the filter is traced continuously by the feedback tone. In the integrate mode less feedback occurs because only the peaks of the filtered wave forming over a period of time triggers the tone. Another feature of the feedback tone is that it can be frequency modulated (FM) to respond to the speed of the brain wave or amplitude modulated (AM) to respond to the height of the wave, or adjusted to respond to a combination of AM and FM.

After building, refinements to the circuit are necessary, such as balancing the gains on the amplifier, to make them equal by adjusting potentiometer settings and passing known voltages for measurement through the circuit. Reference to more technical resources will be necessary in order to put the EEG feedback device into successful operation.

Be assured that this is an excellent circuit and will produce a machine fully competitive with expensive and sophisticated models available on the commercial market. It is suitable for research, meditation or general brain wave biofeedback experimentation. Good luck in your explorations!

BIBLIOGRAPHY

ALBINO, R., AND G. BURNAND, "Continuing of the alpha rhythm in man." *Journal of Experimental Psychology*, Vol. 67 (1964) pp 539–544.

"Alpha Waves of the future." *Time*, Vol. 98 (July 19, 1971), p 33.

ANAND, B.K., G. CHHINA, AND B. BALDEV SINGH, "Some aspects of electroencephalographic studies in Yogis." *Electroencephalography and Clinical Neurophysiology*, Vol. 13 (1961), pp 452–456.

"A Psychophysiological study of out-of-the-body experiences in selected subject." *Journal of the American Society for Psychical Research*, Vol. 62 (1968), pp 3–27.

ALTERMAN, M.B., R.C. HOWES, AND L.R. MACDONALD, "Facilitation of spindle-burst sleep by conditioning of electroencephalographic activity, while awake." *Science*, Vol. 167 (1970), pp 1146–1148.

BAGCHI, B., AND M. WENGER, "Electrophysiological correlates of some Yogi exercises." *Electroencephalography and Clinical Neurophysiology*, Supplement 7 (1957), pp 132–149.

BARBER, T.X., L. DiCARA, J. KAMIYA, N.E. MILLER, D. SHAPIRO, AND J. STOYVA, eds., *Biofeedback and Self Control, 1970: An Aldine Annual on the Regulation of Bodily Processes and Consciousness*. Chicago: Aldine-Atherton, 1971.

BARRAT, P., AND J. HERD, "Subliminal conditioning of alpha rhythm." *Australian Journal of Psychology*, Vol. 16 (1964), pp 9–19.

Bartley, S.C., "The relation between cortical responses to visual stimulation and changes in the alpha rhythm." *Journal of Experimental Psychology*, Vol. 27 (1940), pp 627–639.

BASH, K.W., "The alpha rhythm during relaxed wakefulness, dreams and hallucinations, twilight states and psychoses." *Psychiatric Clinic*, Vol. 1 (1968), pp 152–174.

BEATTY, J., "Effects of initial alpha waves abundance and operant training procedures on occipital alpha and beta wave activity." *Psychonomic Science*, Vol. 23 (1971), pp 197–199.

BECKMAN, F., AND M. STEIN, "A note on the relationship between per cent alpha time and efficiency in problem solving." *Journal of Psychology*, Vol. 51 (1961), pp 169–172.

BERKOUT, J., D. WALTER, AND W.R. ADEY, "Alterations of the human electroencephalogram induced by stressful verbal activity." *EEG Clinical Neurophysiology*, Vol. 27 (1969), pp 457–459.

BLACK, A., "The direct control of neural processes by reward and punishment." *American Scientist*, Vol. 59 (1971), pp 236–245.

BROWN, B.B., "Awareness of EEG-subjectivity activity relationships detected within a closed feedback system." *Psychophysiology*, Vol. 7 (1971), pp 451–464.

BUDZYNSKI, T., AND J. STOYVA, *Biofeedback Techniques in Behavior Therapy and Autogenic Training.* Unpublished manuscript, University of Colorado Medical Center, 1971.

CHAPMAN, R., L. CAVONIUS, AND J. ERNEST, "Alpha and kappa EEG activity in eyeless subjects." *Science*, Vol. 171 (March 19, 1971), pp 1159–1160.

CHERTOK, L., AND P. KRAMARZ, "Hypnosis, sleep and electroencephalography." *Journal of Nervous and Mental Diseases*, Vol. 128 (1959), pp 227–238.

CHILDERS, D., AND N. PERRY, "Alpha-like activity in vision." *Brain Research*, Vol. 25 (1971), pp 1–20.

DARROW, C., AND G. GULLICKSON, "The role of brain waves in learning and other integrative functions." *Recent Advances in Biological Psychiatry*, Vol. 61 (1966), pp 20–27.

DEIKMAN, A., "Experimental meditation." *Journal of Nervous and Mental Disease*, Vol. 136 (1963), pp 329–343.

DIAMANT, J., M. DUFEK, J. HOSKOVEC, M. KRISTOF, V. PERAREK, B. ROTH, AND M. VELEK, "An electrocephalographic study of the waking state and hypnosis." *International Journal of Clinical and Experimental Hypnosis*, Vol. 8 (1960), pp 199–212.

DIMOND, S., AND G. BEAUMONT. "Use of two cerebral hemispheres to increase brain capacity." *Nature*, Vol. 227 (1970), pp 1261–1262.

EISENDRATH, R., "The role of grief and fear in the death of kidney transplant patients." *American Journal of Psychiatry*, Vol. 126 (1969), pp 381–387.

ENGSTROM, D., P. LONDON, AND J. HART, "Hypnotic susceptibility increased by EEG alpha training." *Nature*, Vol. 227 (1970), pp 231–243.

FERNANDEZ, H., R. ROBINSON, AND R. TAYLOR, "A device for testing consciousness," *American Journal of EEG Technology*, Vol. 7 (1967), pp 77–78.

FOULKES, D., and G. VOGEL, "Mental activity at sleep onset." *Journal of Abnormal Psychology*, Vol. 70 (1965), pp 231–243.

GIANNITRAPANI, D., "EEG average frequency and intelligence." *Electroencephalography and Clinical Neuropsysiology*, Vol. 27 (1969), pp 480–486.

GLASS, A., "Intensity of attenuation of alpha activity by mental arithmetic in females and males." *Physiology and Behavior*, Vol. 3 (1968).

GOULD, D., "All a matter of brain waves." *New Statesman*, (January 17, 1969), p 77.

GREEN, A.M., E. GREEN, AND E.D. WALTERS, "Voluntary control of internal states: psychological and physiological." *Journal of Transpersonal Psychology*, Vol. 2 (1970), pp 1–28.

GRIM, P., "Anxiety change produced by self-induced muscle tension and by relaxation with respiration feedback." *Behavior Therapy*, Vol. 2 (1971), pp 11–17.

HARDYCK, C., AND L. PETRINOVICH, "Treatment of subvocal speech during reading." *Journal of Reading*, (February 1969), pp 361–368.

HART, J., "Autocontrol of EEG alpha." *Psychophysiology*, Vol. 4 (1968), p 506.

HEADRICK, M., B. FEATHER, AND D. WELLS, "Unidirectional and large magnitude heart rate changes and augmented sensory feedback." *Psychophysiology*, Vol. 8 (1971), pp 132–142.

HIRAI, T., "Electroencephalographic study on the Zen meditation." *Psychiatria et Neurologia Japonica*, Vol. 62 (1960), pp 76–105.

Honorton, C., "Relationship between EEG alpha activity and ESP card-guessing performance." *Journal of the American Society for Psychical Research*, Vol. 63 (1969), pp 365–374.

"How much for your alpha machine?" *Behavior Today*, September 20, 1971).

"Human Medicine," *Behavior Today*, (May 31, 1971).

JACOBS, A., AND G. FELTON. "Visual feedback of myoelectric output to facilitate muscle relaxation in normal persons and patients with neck injuries." *Archives of Physical Medicine and Rehabilitation*, Vol. 50 (1969), pp 34–39.

KAMIYA, J., "Conscious control of brain waves." *Psychology Today*, Vol. 1 (1968) pp 56–60.

KASAMATSU, A., AND T. HIRAI, "An electroencephalographic study on the Zen meditation (Zazen)," in *Altered States of Consciousness*, C. Tart, ed. New York: Doubleday, 1972.

KASAMATSU, A., T. OKEIMA, S. TAKENAKA, E. KOGA, K. IKEDA, AND H. SUGIYAMA, "The EEG of Zen and Yoga practitioners." *EEG Clinical Neurophysiology*, Vol. 9, (1957), pp 51–52. Supplement.

KREITMAN, N., AND J.C. SHAW, "Experimental enhancement of alpha activity." *EEG Clinical Neurophysiology*, Vol. 18 (1965), pp 147–155.

KRIPPNER, S., AND M. ULLMAN, "Telepathy and dreams: a controlled experiment with electroencephalogram-electro-oculogram monitoring." *Journal of Nervous and Mental Disease*, Vol. 151 (1970), pp. 394–403.

LEVENET, H., B. ENGEL, AND J. PEARSON, "Differential operant conditioning of heart rate." *Psychosomatic Medicine*, Vol. 30 (1968), pp 837–845.

LOOMIS, A.L., E.N. HARVEY, AND G. HOBART, "Brain potentials during hypnosis." *Science*, Vol. 83 (1936), pp. 239–241.

LUBIN, A., L. JOHNSON, AND M. AUSTIN, "Discrimination among states of consciousness using EEG spectra." *Psychophysiology*, Vol. 6 (1969), pp 122–132.

MILLER, H., "Alpha waves—artifacts?" *Psychological Bulletin*, Vol. 69 (1968), pp 279–280.

NOWLIS, D., AND J. KAMIYA, "The control of electroencephalographic alpha rhythms through auditory feedback and the associated mental activity." *Psychophysiology*, Vol. 6 (1970), pp 476–484.

OKEIMA, T., E. KOGU, K. IDEDA, AND H. SUGIYAMA, "The EEG of Yoga and Zen practitioners." *Electroencephalography and Clinical Neurophysiology*, Supplement 9 (1957), p 51.

O'LEARY, J., "Discoverer of the brain wave." *Science*, Vol. 168 (1970), pp 562–563.

OSTRANDER, S., AND L. SCHROEDER, *Psychic Discoveries Behind the Iron Curtain*. Englewood Cliffs, N.J.: Prentice-Hall, 1970.

PASEKEWITZ, D., J. LYNCH, M. ORNE, AND J. COSTELLO, "The Feedback Control of alpha activity: Conditioning or disinhibition?" *Psychophysiology*, Vol. 6 (1970), pp 637–638.

PASSERINI, D., AND S. PATERSON, "A study of cardiac conditioning in man." *Conditional Reflex*, Vol. 1 (1966), pp 90–103.

RAZRAN, G., "The observable unconscious and the inferable conscious in current Soviet psychophysiology: Interoceptive conditioning, semantic conditioning and the orienting reflex." *Psychological Review*, Vol. 68 (1961), pp 81–147.

SCHMEIDLER, G., "High ESP scores after a swami's brief instruction in meditation and breathing." *Journal of the American Society for Psychical Research*, Vol. 64 (1970), pp 100–103.

SHIPMAN, W., D. OKEN, AND H. HEATH, "Muscle tension and effort at self-control during anxiety." *Archives of General Psychiatry*, Vol. 23 (1970), pp 359–368.

SIMPSON, H., A. PAIVIO, AND T. ROGERTS,"Occipital alpha activity of high and low visual imagers during problem solving." *Psychonomic Science*, Vol. 8 (1967), pp 49–50.

SLATER, K., "Alpha rhythms and mental imagery." *Electroencephalography and Clinical Neurophysiology*, Vol. 12 (1960), pp 851–859.

SMART, A., "Conscious control of physical and mental states." *Menninger Perspective*, (April-May 1970).

SPILKER, B., J. KAMIYA, E. CALLAWAY, AND C. YEAGER,"Visual evoked responses in subjects trained to control alpha rhythms." *Psychophysiology*, Vol. 5 (1969), pp 683–695.

STANFORD, R., AND C. LOVIN, "The EEG alpha rhythm and ESP performance." *Journal of the American Society for Psychical Research*, (1970), p 64.

STERMAN, M., "Effects of instrumental EEG conditioning upon sleep and seizure behavior in the cat." *Conditional Reflex*, Vol. 5 (1970), p 185.

TART, C., ed., *Altered States of Consciousness.* New York: Wiley, 1969.

TRAVIS, L.E., AND J.P. EGAN, "Increase in the frequency of the alpha rhythm by verbal stimulation." *Journal of Experimental Psychology*, Vol. 23 (1968), pp. 385–393.

ULLMAN, M., S. KRIPPNER, AND S. FELDSTEIN, "Experimentally induced telepathic dreams: two studies using EEG-Rem monitoring technique." *International Journal of Neuropsychiatry*, Vol. 2 (1966), pp 420–437.

VOGEL, W., D. BROVERMAN, AND E. KLAIBER, "EEG and mental abilities." *Electroencephalography and Clinical Neurophysiology*, Vol. 24 (1968), pp 166–175.

WALLACE, R., "Physiological effects of transcendental meditation." *Science*, Vol. 167 (1970), pp 1751–1754.

WALTER, D., J. RHODES, AND W. ADEY, "Discriminating among states of consciousness by EEG measurements. A study of four subjects." *Electroencephalography and Clinical Neurophysiology*, Vol. 22 (1967), pp 2–29.

WEINER, H., "Current status and future prospects for research in psychosomatic medicine." *Journal of Psychiatric Research*, Vol. 8 (1971), pp 479–498.

Alcoholism, 5
Alma, Sister Mary, 69-70
Alpha (brain waves), 1, 2, 3,
    4-5, 6, 7, 9-10, 11, 12,
    13, 15, 19, 20-21, 23,
    24-26, 27, 28, 29, 35, 38,
    42, 45, 49-50, 51, 52, 59,
    60, 63, 64, 65, 66-67,
    69-76, 78, 81, 83, 100
Altered states of conscious-
    ness, *see* Consciousness
Amphetamines, 49
Anger, 44
Anxiety, 5, 20, 21, 44, 51,
    59, 61, 62, 75, 86
Asthma, 5, 44
Astrology, 29, 40, 41
Awareness, 8, 21, 23, 26,
    28, 29, 34, 35, 68, 71, 72,
    73-76

Behavior modification, 58,
    60
Berger, Hans, 9
Beta brain waves, 12-13,
    18, 19, 59, 100
Biofeedback, 3, 4, 5, 20, 21,
    45, 47, 48, 49, 50, 51, 52,
    53, 54, 57, 58, 59, 60, 61,
    62, 63, 65, 71, 75, 78,
    79-82, 86, 93, 100
Black magic, *see* Occult
Blood pressure, 2, 44, 46,
    47, 54
Brain, 7-9, 10, 12, 19, 20,
    24, 25, 49

Brain waves, 1, 2, 3, 4, 7, 9,
    11, 12, 13, 14-18, 19, 22,
    52, 54, 55, 59, 64, 84, 85,
    101
Brown, Barbara, 12, 24, 54
Buddhist, 2, 42, 65, 66
Burns, Frank, 58-62

Cancer, 5, 46-47
Cardiac problems, *see* Heart
    problems
Circulatory system, 46, 47
Clarke, Arthur C., 42
Colitis, 48, 51
Consciousness, 5, 11, 13, 38
Constipation, 5
Cox, Harvey, 40
Crane, Shirley, 71-72
Creativity, 2, 23, 74-75

Defense Department, 3, 6,
    44 (Pentagon)
Delta brain waves, 12, 16,
    19, 59
Depression, 5
Diarrhea, 48
Drug addiction, 5, 54
Drug coma, 11
Drugs, 13, 23, 28, 29, 30,
    32, 36, 37-39, 47, 53, 66,
    68, 71

Ecstasy, *see* Euphoria
Electrical activity, 1, 7, 8, 9, 10, 12, 14, 19, 24, 49, 85
Electrodes, 9, 10, 11, 14, 19, 20, 24, 25, 50, 51, 52, 72, 81, 82, 83, 93
Electroencephalograph (EEG), 9-11, 12, 13, 14-18, 19, 49, 52, 66, 67, 70, 81-82, 93, 101
Encephalitis, 11
Encounter, 28, 29, 34-36, 60
Epilepsy, 11, 19, 24
Euphoria, 5, 7, 23, 38, 76
Extrasensory perception (ESP), 3, 64, 69-70

Feedback, *see* Biofeedback
Food and Drug Administration, 80
Fornason, Kathleen, 72-73
Freud, Sigmund, 28, 33
Frigidity, 51, 62
Frustration, 45, 60, 62

Galvani, Luigi, 8
Galvanic skin response, 58, 81, 85-93
Gamma brain waves, 13, 19
God, 39, 69

Hare Krishna, 29, 39
Headaches, 5, 24, 47, 53
Healing, 5
Heart problems, 4, 5, 43, 46
Heart rates, 2, 4, 14, 24, 44, 45, 47, 59
Heredity, 13
High blood pressure, *see* Blood pressure
Hoadley, Silas, 66-68
Homosexual, 60
Hyperactivity, 5, 49
Hypertension, 5, 51
Hypnosis, 69, 76
Hypothalamus, 19

I Ching, 40, 41
Impotence, 51, 61
Infectious disease, 44
Insomnia, 5, 52
Intestinal reactions, 47

Kamiya, Joseph, 4, 29, 65, 66-67
Kappa brain waves, 13
King, Martin Luther, 31

Learning, 2, 20, 47, 49, 51
Leary, Timothy, 38
LSD, 38, 80

Machines (brain wave), 3, 4, 9–11, 13, 20–21, 22–26, 35, 38, 42, 50–51, 52, 58, 65, 67, 74–76, 78, 79–101
Marijuana, 4, 30, 80
Martin Marietta Corporation, 3
Meditation, 2, 3, 7, 12, 22, 29, 63, 65–68
Memory, 8
Metabolism, 2
Migraine, 53
Mind control, 69–70
Multiple sclerosis, 5
Muscle tension, *see* Tension

Palmistry, 40
Pavlovian method, 48
Phobias, 51, 80
Pregnancy, 61
Primal therapy, 36, 51
Problem solving, 2, 12
Psychograma, 36
Psychology, 5, 33, 36, 37, 64, 75
Psychophysiological Research, Society for, 79–80
Psychosis, 55
Psychosomatic disease, 44
Psychotherapy, 23, 76

Nall, Angie, 49
Navy, U.S., 52
Needleman, Jacob, 41
Nelson, Bob, 76
Neminski, 9
Nerve cells, 8, 19
Nerve function, 9
Nervous system, 8, 19, 65
Neurosis, 55
Noogenesis, 57–62

Reading, 48–49
Relaxation, *see* Alpha
Religion, 6, 31, 39, 41, 42, 63, 69–70
Rock (music), 29
Roszak, Theodore, 27, 31
Rugh, John D., 85

Obesity, 5
Occult, 40–41, 44, 45
Operant conditioning, 21

Schwitzgebel, Robert L., 84–85
Self, 22
Self-awareness, *see* Awareness
Self-knowledge, *see* Awareness

Sensitivity, *see* Awareness
Sexual problems, 5, 80
Sleep, 12, 13, 23
Stafford, Emerson, 64
Stomach trouble, 47
Stress, 44, 47, 53, 54, 61
Stroke, 5, 11, 46
Sturgis, Norman, 73–76
Stuttering, 5, 49
Surgery, 10
Synanon, 28, 29, 36

Tarot, 40
Tension, 3, 5, 25, 49, 50,
    51–52, 53, 54, 59, 61, 76,
    86
Theta brain waves, 12, 17,
    59, 75, 83, 100
Tranquilizers, 49, 54
Transactional analysis, 28
Tumors (brain), 11, 19, 46

Ulcers, 5, 44

Visual images, 19
Voltaire, Francois, 39
Voodoo, *see* Occult

Warts, 5
Witchcraft, *see* Occult

Xerox Corporation, 3

Yoga, 29, 48

Zen, 3, 5, 12, 22, 28, 42, 64,
    65, 66–68, 69

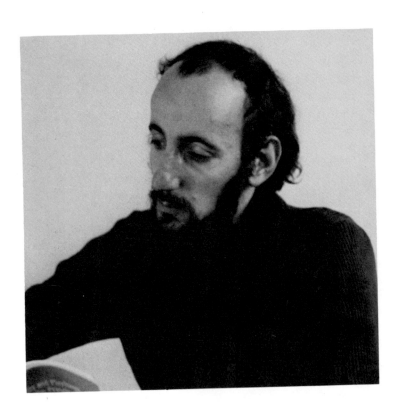

DAVID S. BOXERMAN

A psychiatric social worker for community mental health centers in San Francisco, David Boxerman is daily involved with people who need tranquility and inner calm. For six years he has searched for and examined different modes of therapy for alternatives to the more traditional modes. Biofeedback and alpha brain waves have been found viable and useful.

Born in Jacksonville, Florida, Boxerman is a graduate of San Francisco State University and received his M.S.W. from the University of Missouri. In addition to many leisure time pursuits he is cartoonist for a nationally syndicated weekly cartoon series called *Aleph-Bits*.

David Boxerman, his wife Yvonne and son Aaron, live in Northern California.

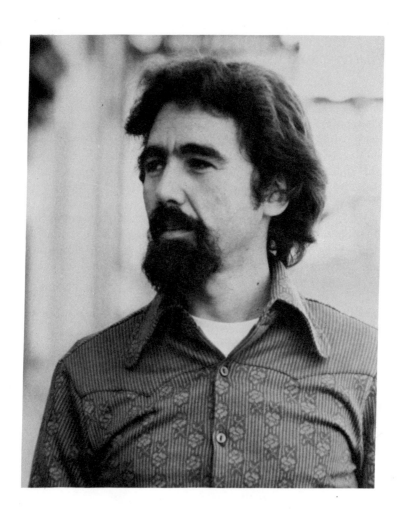

ARON Z. SPILKEN

Presently serving as president of the board of the California Association for Children with Communication Disorders, Aron Spilken works as a psychotherapist in San Francisco's community mental health program. During the past ten years he has divided his time between research and clinical practice, and his professional writing has focused on the relationship between stress and illness.

Born in New London, Connecticut, he is a graduate of Brooklyn College and received his doctorate in psychology from Boston University. He attended the University of Vienna for a year and studied existential psychology under Victor Frankl. He is currently a therapist with the infant stimulation program (therapy with infants with delayed development) in Chinatown, San Francisco.

CELESTIAL ARTS BOOK LIST

LOVE IS AN ATTITUDE, poetry and photographs by Walter Rinder.
03-0 Paper @ $3.95   04-9 Cloth @ $7.95

THIS TIME CALLED LIFE, poetry and photographs by Walter Rinder.
05-7 Paper @ $3.95   06-5 Cloth @ $7.95

SPECTRUM OF LOVE, poetry by Walter Rinder with David Mitchell art.
19-7 Paper @ $2.95   20-0 Cloth @ $7.95

FOLLOW YOUR HEART, poetry by Walter Rinder with Richard Davis art.
39-1 Paper @ $2.95

THE HUMANNESS OF YOU, Vol. 1, art and philosophy by Walter Rinder.
47-2 Paper @ $2.95

THE HUMANNESS OF YOU, Vol. 2, art and philosophy by Walter Rinder.
54-5 Paper @ $2.95

VISIONS OF YOU, poetry by George Betts and photography by Robert Scales.
07-3 Paper @ $3.95

MY GIFT TO YOU, poetry by George Betts and photography by Robert Scales.
15-4 Paper @ $3.95

YOU & I, poetry and photography by Leonard Nimoy.
26-X Paper @ $3.95   27-8 Cloth @ $7.95

WILL I THINK OF YOU?, poetry and photography by Leonard Nimoy.
70-7 Paper @ $3.95

SPEAK THEN OF LOVE, poetry by Andrew Oerke with Asian art.
29-4 Paper @ $3.95

I AM, concepts of awareness in poetic form by Michael Grinder with color art.
25-1 Paper @ $2.95

GAMES STUDENTS PLAY, transactional analysis in schools by Ken Ernst.
16-2 Paper @ $3.95   17-0 Cloth @ $7.95

GUIDE FOR SINGLE PARENTS, transactional analysis by Kathryn Hallett.
55-3 Paper @ $3.95   64-2 Cloth @ $7.95

PASSIONATE MIND, guidance and understanding by Joel Kramer.
63-4 Paper @ $3.95

SENSIBLE BOOK, understanding children's senses by Barbara Polland.
53-7 Paper @ $3.95

THIS TIMELESS MOMENT, Aldous Huxley's life by Laura Huxley.
22-5 Paper @ $4.95

HEALING MIND, explains the healing powers of the mind by Dr. Irving Oyle.
80-4 Paper @ $4.95

HOW TO BE SOMEBODY, a guide for personal growth by Yetta Bernhard.
20-9 Paper @ $4.95

CREATIVE SURVIVAL, the problems of single mothers by Persia Woolley.
17-9 Paper @ $4.95

FAT LIBERATION, the awareness technique to losing weight by Alan Dolit.
03-9 Paper @ $3.95

INWARD JOURNEY, art as therapy by Margaret Keyes.
81-2 Paper @ $4.95

GOD, poetic visions of the abstract by Alan Watts.
75-8 Paper @ $3.95

Write for a free catalog to:
CELESTIAL ARTS   231 Adrian Road   Millbrae, California 94030